CONTACT
LENS
PROBLEM
SOLVING

CONTACT LENS PROBLEM SOLVING

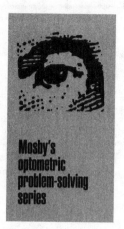

Mosby's optometric problem-solving series

Edited by

Edward S. Bennett
O.D., F.A.A.O.

University of Missouri–St. Louis
School of Optometry
St. Louis, Missouri

Series Editor

Richard London
MA., O.D., F.A.A.O.

Diplomate, Binocular Vision and Perception
Pediatric and Rehabilitative Optometry
Oakland, California

with 40 illustrations and 32 color plates

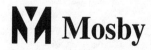 Mosby

St. Louis Baltimore Berlin Boston Carlsbad Chicago London Madrid
Naples New York Philadelphia Sydney Tokyo Toronto

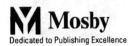

Mosby
Dedicated to Publishing Excellence

Executive Editor: Martha Sasser
Associate Developmental Editor: Kellie F. White
Project Manager: John Rogers
Production Editor: George B. Stericker, Jr.
Designer: Renée Duenow
Manufacturing Supervisor: Betty Richmond
Cover Design: Jason Sonderman

Printed in the United States of America
Composition by Carlisle Communications, Ltd.
Printing/binding by Plus Communications

Mosby–Year Book, Inc.
11830 Westline Industrial Drive
St. Louis, Missouri 63146

Library of Congress Cataloging in Publication Data

Contact lens problem solving / edited by Edward S. Bennett.
     p.   cm. — (Mosby's optometric problem solving series)
    Includes bibliographical references and index.
    ISBN 0-8151-0424-3
    1. Contact lenses.   I. Bennett, Edward S. II. Series.
    [DNLM: 1. Contact Lenses. WW 355 C75575 1995]
RE977.C6C55584 1995
617.7'523—dc20
DNLM/DLC
for Library of Congress   94-19441
                                    · CIP

94 95 96 97 98 / 9 8 7 6 5 4 3 2 1

Contributors

Keith S. Ames, O.D.
Private Practice,
Chillicothe, Ohio

William G. Bachman, O.D., M.S.
Associate Professor,
School of Optometry,
University of Missouri–St. Louis,
St. Louis, Missouri

Larry J. Davis, O.D., F.A.A.O.
Assistant Professor of Optometry,
University of Missouri–St. Louis;
Adjunct Assistant Professor,
Department of Ophthalmology,
St. Louis University School of Medicine,
St. Louis, Missouri

Robert M. Grohe, O.D.
Private Practitioner,
Clinical Associate Professor of
 Ophthalmology,
Northwestern University School
 of Medicine
Chicago, Illinois

Vinita Allee Henry, O.D.
Clinical Associate Professor and
 Co-Chief,
Contact Lens Clinic,
School of Optometry,
University of Missouri–St. Louis,
St. Louis, Missouri

Neelu F. Hira, O.D.
Private Practitioner,
Optometric Resident at Westside VA
 Hospital,
Chicago, Illinois

Patricia M. Keech, O.D.
Assistant Chief, Contact Lens Section,
Group Health Cooperative of Puget
 Sound,
Seattle, Washington

Judith L. Kremer, O.D.
Clinical Assistant Professor,
School of Optometry,
University of Missouri–St. Louis,
St. Louis, Missouri

Ian M. Lane, O.D.

Private Practice,
Anaheim, California

Thomas G. Quinn, O.D., M.S.

Private Practice,
Athens, Ohio

Melvin J. Remba, O.D.

Chief Optometric Clinical Services,
Cedars-Sinai Medical Center,
Los Angeles, California

Cristina M. Schnider, O.D.

Chief, Contact Lens Services,
Pacific University Family Vision Centers;
Associate Professor,
Pacific University College of Optometry,
Forest Grove, Oregon

I dedicate this book to my wife, Jean,
and my children, Matt and Josh,
and to every contact lens practitioner
interested in providing both optimum care
and the most appropriate contact lens materials
for all motivated patients.

E.S.B.

Preface

The purpose of this text is to provide both practitioners and students with a clinical guide intended to serve as a useful reference source in everyday contact lens practice. The text is unique in that its content is exclusively clinical cases. These cases are not rare and unique but address common everyday routine and challenging patient encounters. The format of each chapter not only provides a successful management plan but also discusses other methods of managing the case. Interspersed within these chapters are clinical pearls and fitting techniques intended to upgrade the reader's knowledge in fitting contact lens patients and troubleshooting problems.

Each of the nine chapters included in this text pertains to an important segment of contact lens practice. These include rigid lens fitting, rigid lens care and compliance, hydrogel lens fitting, hydrogel lens care and compliance, disposable lenses, toric fitting, presbyopic fitting, irregular corneas, and management of contact lens–induced complications. The cases are intended to be generic whenever possible and to emphasize the use of a variety of methods and lens materials in their successful management. Although these management plans may not be successful in every case and reflect the individual author's recommendations, they are intended to represent effective solutions to be considered when similar patients are presented in practice.

I would like to acknowledge series editor Dr. Richard London for allowing me to have this opportunity. I would also like to express my appreciation to the staff at Mosby–Year Book, Inc., for their support and assistance. The computer talents of my assistant, Judie Walter, and the input of Jerry Christensen, O.D., Ph.D., Dean of the University of Missouri–St. Louis School of Optometry, are greatly appreciated. Finally, without the tremendous effort by the outstanding group of clinicians who contributed to this text, it would not have been possible. So, in closing, I thank Keith Ames, Gary Bachman, Larry Davis, Bob Grohe, Vinita Henry, Neelu Hira, Pat Keech, Judie Kremer, Ian Lane, Tom Quinn, Mel Remba, and Cristina Schnider.

Ed Bennett

Contents

CONTACT LENS PROBLEM SOLVING

1

Rigid Gas-Permeable Lens Design, Fitting, and Problem Solving

Cristina M. Schnider
Keith S. Ames

The success of a rigid gas permeable lens fit is dependent on many factors, including patient and practitioner motivation, ocular and refractive characteristics, and (perhaps most important) a suitable rigid lens design. Although lens fitting philosophies have changed through the years and may vary considerably from practitioner to practitioner, some basic factors apply if one is to achieve consistent success with this modality. The following cases illustrate some of the basic design principles in terms of selection of lens material, diameter, base curve–cornea relationship, peripheral curve design, and modifications that can be employed in fitting rigid gas-permeable (RGP) lenses.

• Case One: Poor Comfort

I. Subjective Data

A 19-year-old man was initially fitted with RGP contact lenses to correct his moderate myopia and with-the-rule corneal astigmatism. Lenses were dispensed, with the patient noting moderate lens awareness but with excellent vision (20/15 OU). He then was instructed to try wearing the lenses at least 6 to 8 hours the first day, adding 1 or 2 hours per day but not to exceed 12 hours, and to return in 1 week. At the 1 week follow-up visit, he reported that he could not progress beyond 4 hours of wear, after which time his eyes became sore.

II. Objective Data

Visual acuity was confirmed to be 20/15 OD, OS, OU, with a binocularly balanced overrefraction of plano in each eye. The lens fitting relationship appeared to be excellent—with good horizontal and vertical centration, minimal apical clearance, smooth transition zones, and moderately wide edge clearance in primary gaze. Movement was sluggish but unrestricted in all gazes; however, a mild arcuate area of fluorescein pooling was visible in the mid-peripheral superior cornea when the lens was worn. Another arcuate band of conjunctival staining was noted parallel to the inferior limbus. Inspection of the lens on and off the eye revealed no obvious imperfections, and parameters were verified as specified.

III. Assessment/Plan

The arcuate indentation seen superiorly following several blinks indicated a need for more adequate blending of the peripheral curve junctions to allow the lens to move smoothly across the peripheral cornea during the blink cycle. The inferior conjunctival staining represented a consistent pattern of tear film rupture on the inferior lens edge and was attributed to a thick and/or blunt lens edge. To facilitate lens movement and tear exchange, the lens was blended with radius tools approximately halfway between each pair of peripheral curves. After blending, the lens edge was rolled to smooth and round the anterior and posterior surfaces, thereby minimizing disruption of the tear film by the lens edge.

IV. Alternative Management Plan/Summary

The patient reported an immediate increase in comfort following lens modification, and lens movement was observed to be smoother with the blink. A simple modification, such as blending and rolling the edge, creaded vastly improved comfort during the adaptation period of RGP lens wear (Table 1-1).

CLINICAL PEARL

A simple modification, such as blending and rolling the edge, can create vastly improved comfort during the adaptation period of RGP lens wear.

Patients who experience difficulty building up wearing time generally benefit from these modifications. With modern RGP materials having good oxygen transmissibility, there should be no physiological need

TABLE 1-1

Rigid Gas-Permeable Lens Modification Summary

Technique	Equipment	Procedure	Illustration
Blend series	Modification Unit (1000 rpm)	Select radius tool ≥ 1.5 mm flatter than lens base curve and place on modification spindle	
	Brass or Delrin radius tools (8.0, 9.0, 10.0, 11.0, 12.0 mm)		
	Velveteen cloth (untreated)	Wet velveteen and secure over tool with O ring	
	Rubber O rings	Apply polish to velveteen	
	Polishing compound	Affix lens concave side out to suction cup	
	Suction cup lens holder	Using gentle pressure, place lens on tool at slight angle to vertical and rotate one half turn; repeat 6 to 8 times for medium blend, reapplying polish as needed to cool lens	
Edge roll	Modification unit	Wet sponge thoroughly and squeeze gently to remove excess water; place in drum tool on modification unit	
	3-inch drum tool with 1-inch deep firm sponge		
	Polishing compound	Apply polish to sponge	
	Suction cup holder	Mount lens concave size out on suction cup; place in spinner (if available)	
	Spinner desirable	Beginning at 60° angle to sponge in center, roll lens to edge while decreasing angle to 30°	
	Remount lens convex side out and repeat		

for lengthy adaptation periods as were needed with polymethyl methacrylate (PMMA), with which patients had to be "weaned off" oxygen. Additionally, forcing a short wearing time acts as a deterrent to wearing the lenses, since most patients' days are 8 to 10 hours long and earlier removal often means significant interruption of their daily routine. Therefore patients should be encouraged to quickly build up their wearing time (to a maximum of 12 to 15 hours). The main adaptation that must occur concerns the lens-lid interaction and requires smooth surfaces over all the lens. Even when the exact specifications of the posterior lens periphery are not known, selecting a series of two or three velveteen-covered radius tools 1.5 to 3 mm flatter than the base curve radius for blending will usually cause an appreciable increase in lens comfort. Any peripheral modification should be followed by edge rolling, because removing material in the periphery often results in a thinning and sharpening of the lens edge. Using spindle speeds not exceeding 1000 rpm and liberal amounts of lens polish will cause the least insult to the lens material.

• Case Two: Corneal Distortion/Molding

I. Subjective Data

A 25-year-old woman requested that her RGP contact lenses be evaluated because she wished to resume wear after last using them over 2 years earlier. She was getting married in 3 months and did not want to wear her spectacles for the wedding photographs. She had stopped wearing her lenses because of instability of her vision with them and the problems she had had adjusting to glasses following lens wear.

II. Objective Data

Manifest refraction

OD: $-3.25 - 2.50 \times 165$ 20/20
OS: $-2.75 - 2.75 \times 15$ 20/20

Keratometry

OD: 43.00 @ 165; 45.75 @ 75   (smooth mires)
OS: 43.25 @ 015; 46.25 @ 105   (smooth mires)

Lens verification (patient's own)

	BCR	OZD	Power	OAD	CT
OD:	7.67 mm	7.6 mm	−4.25 D	9.0 mm	0.13 mm
OS:	7.67 mm	7.6 mm	−3.50 D	9.0 mm	0.14 mm

Lens assessment (patient's own)

OU: Lenses positioned high, under upper lid, with central pooling and mid-peripheral bearing resembling a double D characteristic of steep fit on moderate to high with-the-rule cornea

Visual acuity with contact lenses

		Over-refraction	
OD:	20/15-	Plano − 0.25 × 90	(20/15)
OS:	20/15-	Plano − 0.50 × 90	(20/15)

The patient was asked to resume wear of her own lenses and to return in 1 week for a follow-up evaluation. At that time she reported good comfort but was also experiencing the same symptoms that had led to her discontinuation of lens wear 2 years previously.

Visual acuity at 1 week

		Over-refraction	
OD:	20/25	+0.50 − 1.00 × 005	(20/15)
OS:	20/20-	+0.75 − 0.75 × 180	(20/15)

Lens assessment

OU: Fluorescein pattern unchanged from that seen at initial visit; marked staining at 3 and 9 o'clock (Plate 1)

Front surface keratometry (FSK) with lenses in place

OD: 41.00 @ 180; 42.50 @ 90   (mire alignment varies with blink)
OS: 39.50 @ 180; 40.75 @ 90   (mire distortion slightly with blink)

Manifest refraction following lens wear

OD: -3.50 − 1.25 × 165   (20/20)
OS: -3.00 − 1.25 × 15   (20/20)

III. Assessment/Plan

The visual instability reported by the patient while wearing lenses was undoubtedly due to lens flexure, as evidenced by the FSK readings and spherocylindrical overrefraction. This amount of flexure is not uncommon with a steeper-than-K fitting relationship on a moderately high with-the-rule cornea. In addition, the corneal molding that takes place when a spherical lens is placed on an astigmatic cornea accounts for the patient's problems with her spectacles following lens wear. The patient was refitted with a 2 D spherical power effect (SPE) bitoric contact lens with an alignment-fitting relationship in the horizontal meridian.

The SPE lens has optical properties of a spherical lens, but fitting properties of a toric lens, and is simply derived from Ks and the spectacle prescription. The back surface is designed to physically correct approximately two thirds of the corneal cylinder, leaving sufficient "rocking" room to allow for adequate tear exchange and smooth lens movement in the vertical meridian. An alignment-fitting relationship minimizes desiccation in the 3 and 9 o'clock areas by facilitating better tear exchange in the horizontal meridian compared to that in a steep relationship. The power of the lens is determined by the fitting relationship (on K) and the amount of back surface toricity (2 D).

Final lens parameters

	BCR	Power	OAD
OD:	7.85/7.50 (43.00/45.00)	−3.25/−5.25	9.0 mm
OS:	7.80/7.46 (43.25/45.25)	−2.75/−4.75	9.0 mm

At the 1 week follow-up visit following dispensing of the bitoric lenses, the patient reported that her vision remained consistently clear with the new lenses and that she no longer experienced problems adapting to her spectacles. The level of peripheral staining had decreased significantly as well.

IV. Alternative Management Plan Summary

A bitoric lens allows the fitter to effectively turn a highly toric cornea into a low with-the-rule astigmat, which is considered ideal for RGP lens fitting. The SPE concept simplifies lens design and eliminates problems associated with toric power rotational effects. Table 1-2 details fitting and optical considerations in fitting the astigmatic patient.

Aspheric rigid lens designs have also been suggested for correcting moderately astigmatic corneas, but even in the presence of a more acceptable fluorescein pattern, corneal molding and resultant spectacle blur still may occur with these designs.

CLINICAL PEARL

A bitoric lens allows the fitter to effectively turn a highly toric cornea into a low with-the-rule astigmat, which is considered to be ideal for RGP lens fitting.

TABLE 1-2

Physical and Optical Considerations for Fitting the Astigmatic Patient

Lens design	Physical indications	Optical indications	Comments
Spherical RGP	Low WTR cornea (≤ 2.00)	K cylinder ~ Refractive cylinder	Increase CT to prevent flexure
Spherical RGP with toric periphery	Moderate WTR or low ATR cornea (1.50 to 2.50)	K cylinder ~ Refractive cylinder	Optical zone will be oval
Aspheric RGP (moderate e value)	Moderate WTR or low ATR cornea (1.50 to 3.00)	K cylinder ~ Refractive cylinder	May require steeper than K fit
Front toric RGP	Low WTR cornea (≤ 2.00)	Residual ATR cylinder	Requires prism ballast and/or truncation for stability
Bitoric RGP	High WTR or moderate ATR cornea	SPE: K cylinder ~ Refractive cylinder CPE: K cylinder ≠ Refractive cylinder	Spherical peripheral curves create oval optical zone

WTR, ATR, With and against the rule; SPE, CPE, spherical and cylindrical power effect; CT, center thickness.

• Case Three: Corneal Desiccation

I. Subjective Data

A 32-year-old woman complained of decreased wearing time over the past few months accompanied by marked redness in the temporal quadrant of each eye after 2 to 3 hours of lens wear. She had worn PMMA lenses for 15 years before being switched to RGP lenses the previous year by her former practitioner.

II. Objective Data

Visual acuity was recorded as 20/20 OU with a binocularly balanced over-refraction of plano in each eye. Evaluation of the lens fitting relationship revealed a lens which appeared much too large for the patient's cornea, with a "bulls-eye" fluorescein pattern: central alignment surrounded by a ring of pooling, followed by a ring of mid-peripheral bearing, and a narrow band of edge pooling in the horizontal meridian (Plate 2). Coalesced patches of grade 2+ staining were evident nasally on each cornea, with heavier staining noted temporally in each eye. White light observation revealed infiltration and hyperplasia of the temporal corneas in each eye, with markedly dilated limbal and conjunctival vessels in the area.

III. Assessment/Plan

A diagnosis of 3 and 9 o'clock staining with early vascularized limbal keratitis (VLK) was made, presumably secondary to refitting with a large-diameter low–edge lift lens. Due to the relatively early stages of the VLK, the patient was refitted with a smaller-diameter lens with moderate edge lift and continued wearing this with the addition of antioxidant lubricant qid. After 2 weeks she reported vastly improved comfort, decreased hyperemia, and increased wear time. However, the hypertrophy and infiltration did not completely clear for another 2 weeks, and she was then instructed to continue using the antioxidant drops two to three times per day whenever she wore her lenses and to limit her wearing time to 12 to 14 hours per day.

IV. Alternative Management Plan/Summary

The management of 3 and 9 o'clock staining (which can lead to more advanced problems, such as VLK) is concerned primarily with assuring adequate tear exchange. Historically the concern was over continuity of the anterior tear film, with recommendations made to reduce edge lift and edge thickness. However, with contemporary lens designs that are larger and have lower edge lifts than older PMMA designs, the concern is with tear exchange underneath the lens. Lens diameter should be small enough to allow unrestricted movement of the lens in lateral gaze but large enough to prevent flare from the optical zone junction in lower light conditions. The peripheral curves must be sufficiently flat and wide to allow a peripheral reservoir of tears 0.3 to 0.4 mm in width of vivid green with fluorescein but not so flat as to cause a negative meniscus, or black line formation, at the lens edge. Blends should also be moderate to allow smooth movement and unrestricted tear flow behind the lens.

Vascularized limbal keratitis is an extreme result of inattention to these design rules. It is characterized by chronic peripheral corneal desiccation, which results in irritation and dilation of the limbal arcade, and ultimately leads to infiltration of the peripheral cornea. In later stages epithelial hypertrophy results, creating further disruption of the tear film and vascularization increases following continued insult. The main factor associated with VLK appears to be large-diameter lenses with low edge lift, which cause mechanical chafing leading to insufficient tear flow over the peripheral cornea. The reported association with previous PMMA lens wear may, in fact, be coincidental, since the overwhelming tendency when refitting PMMA patients is to increase the lens diameter. In early cases, simply decreasing the diameter and increasing the edge lift may be sufficient to solve the problem. Later stages often require a period of no lens wear and even steroids to quiet the response before refitting with a more appropriate design.

• Case Four: RGP Lens Adherence

I. Subjective Data

A 25-year-old man presented for routine aftercare following 9 months of RGP lens wear. He had no complaints and appeared to have been following his prescribed care and wearing schedule.

II. Objective Data

Entering visual acuity

		Over-refraction	
OD:	20/20	Plano	(20/20)
OS:	20/20−	+0.25	(20/20)

Lens assessment

OD: Centered, positioned slightly under upper lid; apical alignment with optimal edge lift and blends and smooth adequate movement on the blink

OS: Lens adherent, with bubbles trapped under inferior edge and mucus trapped in mid-periphery

Biomicroscopy with lenses removed

OD: Mild 3 and 9 o'clock punctate staining, with diffuse superficial punctate keratitis covering entire cornea; tear film stable

OS: Moderate central punctate staining with diffuse superficial punctate keratitis over remainder of cornea and "strand of pearls" denoting location of trapped bubbles; indentation ring visible with tear film breakup over area of indentation (Plate 3)

Keratometry

OD: 43.50 @ 180; 45.00 @ 90 (smooth mires)
OS: 43.75 @ 180; 44.00 @ 90 (mires mildly distorted)

Manifest refraction

OD: −3.00 −1.00 × 180   20/20
OS: −2.50 −0.75 × 160   20/25−

Additional history

Upon further questioning, the patient remembered that his lenses had been more difficult to remove over the past few months than when he had first gotten them. Review of his record indicated that he had been given Boston solutions but did not specify Boston Original or Boston Advance. The patient identified the Advance solution as the one he was currently using and said it was what he had been given at his previous visit.

The patient was asked to leave both lenses off for a full day, and was given Boston Original conditioner to replace the Advance solution. He returned after 1 week with improved vision and comfort and a stable refraction in both eyes, which gave him 20/20 acuities with and without lenses. The lenses fitted well and moved adequately, with only a trace of 3 and 9 o'clock staining evident. The patient reported no more problems with lens removal and said that he noticed both increased comfort and decreased mucus strands while wearing the lenses.

III. Assessment/Plan

The lens adherence was thought to be due to a mild keratitis caused by reaction to the Boston Advance conditioning solution and the increase in mucus production that typically occurs with corneal irritation.

The primary factor in RGP lens adherence is thought to be a mucus adhesion phenomenon, often with a decrease in aqueous tear film between lens and cornea. In this case, since the fit was acceptable in the nonadherent eye and lens wear had been without incident for the first 6 months, the solution change was deemed sufficient as a first attempt to solve the problem.

IV. Alternative Management Plan/Summary

The mucus adhesion phenomenon has been well documented in extended wear, and the clinical characteristics observed in daily wear patients support this mechanism. Since the related finding of decreased aqueous volume is also present in some adherence cases, strategies to improve tear volume under the lens may also be necessary to correct the problem. If no evidence of solution reaction is present or if changing the solution system is not sufficient to eliminate the adherence, additional steps must be taken. Blending the peripheral curve system will often assist in the exchange of tear volume from beneath the lens, allowing the replenishment of aqueous with each blink. Lens design changes that may be helpful include reducing the diameter, increasing the edge clearance and refitting to achieve minimal apical clearance.

CLINICAL PEARL

A smaller lens diameter with slight apical clearance, good blends, and moderate edge lift allows sufficient tear volume to separate the lens from the mucus layer, thus preventing the contact necessary to bring about lens adherence.

A smaller lens diameter with slight apical clearance, good blends, and moderate edge lift allows sufficient tear volume to separate the lens from the mucus layer, thus preventing the contact necessary to bring about lens adherence.

• Case Five: Variable Vision and Flare

I. Subjective Data

A 38-year-old man presented with complaints of variable vision with his contact lenses, especially at night. He also reported that the headlights of oncoming traffic caused an uncomfortable glare. He had worn hydrogel lenses previously but was refitted into his current RGP correction approximately 3 years ago to "correct his astigmatism." Lens comfort was good although he occasionally had difficulty removing the lenses.

II. Objective Data

Keratometry

OD: 45.75 @ 180; 47.00 @ 90 (smooth mires)
OS: 45.75 @ 180; 47.00 @ 90 (smooth mires)

Manifest refraction

OD: −6.00 −1.50 × 180
OS: −7.00 −1.25 × 180

Contact lens parameters

	OAD	BCR	Power	Material
OD:	9.5 mm	7.45 mm	−5.50 D	Boston 4
OS:	9.5 mm	7.45 mm	−6.25 D	Boston 4

Tricurve design

Lens fit and appearance

Both lenses were positioned very high, with the upper edge of each extending beyond the superior limbus. The patient's upper lids were tight and attached to the lenses forcefully with each blink. The lenses appeared to be aligned centrally but excessive edge lift was noted. The edge of the optical zone was just at the inferior pupil margin.

Biomicroscopy

No corneal edema or staining was present. However, upon lens removal, an arcuate impression line was noted in the superior conjunctiva of both eyes coincident with the upper edge of the lens.

Visual acuity with contact lenses

OD: 20/20
OS: 20/20

III. Assessment/Plan

Excessive superior RGP decentration can cause several clinical problems. Visual performance is often compromised because the patient is looking through the peripheral optics of the lens and the resultant refractive power and junctional zones can interfere with visual acuity. Physiological problems can also result as excessive pressure is applied to the superior corneal/limbal region. Superior limbal keratoconjunctivitis, corneal distortion, and scarring are possible. Intermittent lens adherence is also occasionally observed in this situation.

Refitting the patient into a larger-diameter lens could potentially solve the visual fluctuation/flare complaints but would only compound the lens-positioning problem. With his tight upper lids and high minus refractive error, a larger lens would only attach to the upper lids more strongly and decenter more superiorly. Clearly a different solution was required.

He was refitted into larger-diameter Boston Envision aspheric lenses. The new parameters were

	OAD	BCR	Power	Material
OD:	9.9 mm	7.40 mm	−5.50 D	Boston RXD
OS:	9.9 mm	7.40 mm	−6.25 D	Boston RXD

IV. Alternative Management Plan/Summary

The Envision lens was chosen for several reasons. Research has shown that aspheric designs have less tendency to decenter vertically maintaining a more centered position on the eye. In addition, aspherical designs, like the Boston Envision, have no distinct junctional areas in the periphery that can interfere with visual performance. Plates 4 and 5 compare a typical multicurve spherical with an aspherical design. Note that, even after blending, the spherical lens has a distinct peripheral junction but the aspheric design is free of any discernible junctional areas. Finally, aspheric designs enhance the use of larger diameters. Gradual flattening in the lens midperiphery permits cornea/lens alignment without excessive edge lift.

The Boston Envision lenses did fit this patient as predicted and decentered less superiorly. A recheck 1 month later found him to be satisfied with the new lenses. They were as comfortable as the original ones, with increased stability of vision and decreased flare noted.

Variable vision associated with lens positioning and/or design is not uncommon. Although most RGP lens wearers experience clear and stable vision, problems can result if the peripheral zones of a lens impinge on the visual axis through either excessive decentering or a small overall or optical zone diameter (or a combination of the two). Research has shown that of all the possible factors involved in RGP fitting (including design, fitting relationship, and material), overall diameter has the greatest impact on visual stability. A 9.5 mm diameter lens provides significantly greater visual stability on average than a 9.0 mm diameter lens. A previous hydrogel lens wearer such as this man is even more likely to notice variable vision since soft lens acuity, though not always optimal, is reasonably consistent. Working within an overall diameter range of 9.3 to 9.9 mm and minimizing excessive decentration will help promote clear and stable vision for RGP wearers. The box lists several approaches that can be taken if variable vision due to excessive superior positioning is noted.

CLINICAL PEARL

Research has shown that aspheric designs have less tendency to decenter vertically, maintaining a more centered position on the eye. In addition, aspherical designs, like the Boston Envision, have no distinct junctional areas in the periphery that can interfere with visual performance.

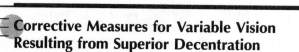

Corrective Measures for Variable Vision Resulting from Superior Decentration

Extend optics of lens beyond the pupil
   Increase overall diameter
   Increase optic zone diameter
Promote a more centered fit
   Thinner edge design (lenticulation)
   Steeper base curve/peripheral curves
   Aspheric design
Increase lens weight
   Increase the center thickness
   Refit into heavier material (such as fluoro-silicone/acrylate)
   Prism ballast
Combinations of the above

• Case Six: Inferior Decentration

I. Subjective Data

A 40-year-old woman presented for her routine eye examination wearing rigid gas-permeable (RGP) lenses that had been fitted approximately 5 years earlier by another practitioner. Before that she had worn PMMA (polymethyl methacrylate) lenses successfully for about 20 years. Her previous practitioner had recommended refitting into RGP lenses to "improve eye health." Although she was generally satisfied with her current contact lens correction, she did have several minor complaints: Her eyes felt dry and burned especially at the end of the day, and there was an occasional slight lens awareness that she had not had with her previous lenses.

II. Objective Data

Keratometry

OD: 43.00 @ 180; 44.25 @ 090 (smooth mires)
OS: 43.50 @ 005; 44.50 @ 095 (smooth mires)

Manifest refraction

OD: $-3.50 -1.00 \times 180$
OS: $-4.00 -0.75 \times 10$

Contact lens parameters

	OAD	BCR	Power	Material
OD:	9.0 mm	7.76 mm	-3.75 D	Boston 2
OS:	9.0 mm	7.76 mm	-4.00 D	Boston 2

Tricurve design

Lens fit and appearance

Both lenses were positioned slightly inferior to the center and appeared to be steep centrally, especially the right lens. Peripheral clearance was minimal, as was lens movement, and partial blinking was occasionally observed.

Biomicroscopy

No corneal edema was present. Light punctate staining was observed in the 3- and 9-o'clock corneal region adjacent to the lens edge in both eyes.

Visual acuity with contact lenses

OD: 20/20–
OS: 20/20

III. Assessment/Plan

We see patients like this individual quite often. They are successfully wearing RGP lenses but are not entirely happy with their correction.

Often their complaints are vague and dismissed by the practitioner. In this case the previous practitioner made the correct recommendation to refit into an RGP material but did not take advantage of the refitting to "fine tune" the fitting characteristics of the lenses.

We were fortunate to have access to the original PMMA lenses (she kept them as spares, as is often the case) and determined that the previous practitioner had simply duplicated the PMMA parameters. There is merit to this approach, especially when selecting the appropriate base curve radius and power for a distorted cornea. However, the fitting characteristics of the original lenses should be carefully evaluated and minor parameter changes considered to optimize fitting of the new lenses and to take advantage of improved material performance.

The patient was refitted with lenses that were slightly larger and flatter than her current correction. The new parameters were

	OAD	BCR	Power	Material
OD:	9.5 mm	7.94 mm	−3.00 D	Boston 2
OS:	9.5 mm	7.85 mm	−3.50 D	Boston 2

Tricurve design

The lenses now showed a central alignment relationship, moderate edge lift, superior positioning, and smooth movement (with the upper lens edge tucked slightly under the upper lid). A recheck approximately 1 month later showed her symptoms to be significantly reduced and no corneal staining evident. She was very pleased with the new lenses.

IV. Alternative Management Plan/Summary

There are two important lessons here. Do not be afraid to make minor RGP parameter changes, even with "successful" contact lens wearers, if you feel fitting performance can be optimized. Remember that RGP fitting is usually quite logical and predictable; minor diameter and base curve radius adjustments within a given design can noticeably improve lens positioning and movement characteristics for enhanced performance.

This patient represented a rather straightforward application of these principles, experiencing better comfort and improved corneal physiology through a more superiorly positioned lens that moved freely with blinking. Other patients will be more challenging, presenting with more severe signs and symptoms, but the principles remain the same: superior positioning, central alignment, and a lens that moves with the upper lid.

Table 1-3 provides guidelines for initial lens selection, and the box lists suggested parameter changes for a given design when lens positioning is a problem. Remember: These guidelines apply to conventional multicurve spherical designs with progressively flatter

TABLE 1-3
Initial Lens Selection

Corneal toricity	Lens diameter		
(D)	9.3	9.6	9.9
0 to 1.00	0.25 flat to On K	0.75 to 0.50 flat	1.00 to 0.75 flat
1.25 to 2.00	On K to 0.25 steep	0.50 to 0.25 flat	0.75 to 0.50 flat
2.25 to 3.00	0.25 to 0.50 steep	0.25 flat to On K	0.50 to 0.25 flat
Greater than 3.00		Consider toric designs	

peripheral curves. Fitting principles for certain aspherical and specialty designs may differ.

Suggested Parameter Changes When Inferior Decentration is a Problem

When the upper lid covers the superior limbus	When the upper lid does not cover the superior limbus
Larger diameter	Smaller diameter
Flatter base curve	Steeper base curve
Thinner overall lens design	Thinner overall lens design
Lighter material	Lighter material
Minus carrier lenticulation for plus powers	Aspheric designs

• Case Seven: Poor Visual Acuity

I. Subjective Data

A 32-year-old woman presented with complaints of poor visual acuity in one eye for about a month. She was a long-term RGP lens wearer but had recently been refitted in our office. Approximately 6 months earlier she had come to our clinic complaining of reduced wearing time, dirty filmy lenses, and a slight discharge. Attempts by previous practitioners to alter care systems and wearing schedules had failed to solve these problems. She had presented at that time with moderately coated silicone/acrylate RGP lenses and 3+ giant papillary conjunctivitis (GPC) in each eye. I recommended refitting with fluoro-silicone/acrylate lenses, which in my experience have less tendency for protein deposition. Follow-up visits showed clean lens surfaces and a reduction in subjective complaints and objective signs. However, visual acuity was definitely reduced in one eye.

CLINICAL PEARL

Refitting giant papillary conjunctivitis patients with fluorosilicone/acrylate materials can be helpful because these materials have less tendency for protein deposition.

II. Objective Data

Keratometry

OD: 44.00 @ 010; 45.00 @ 100 (smooth mires)
OS: 43.75 @ 175; 44.50 @ 085 (smooth mires)

Manifest refraction

OD: −3.00 −1.25 × 005
OS: −3.00 −1.00 × 180

Contact lens parameters

	OAD	BCR	CT	Power
OD:	9.6 mm	7.75 mm	0.15 mm	−2.75 D
OS:	9.6 mm	7.75 mm	0.15 mm	−2.75 D

Fluoroperm 30 material

Lens fit and appearance

Both lenses were positioned somewhat superiorly under the upper lids. Central alignment and moderate edge lift were noted. Movement was smooth with the blink. Lens surfaces were clean and wetted well.

Biomicroscopy

Grade 2 GPC OU and grade 1 limbal injection OU were noted. The corneas were clear, with no staining observed.

Visual acuity with contact lenses

OD: 20/20
OS: 20/25

Lens inspection

Lens powers were verified to be as ordered. The right lens base curve was correct and undistorted. However, the left lens base curve was distorted showing approximately 0.06 mm of toricity.

III. Assessment/Plan

This patient's left lens was warped and appeared to be the most likely explanation for her visual problems. The blurred vision she reported in the left eye was of recent onset (not observed at dispensing or subsequent rechecks) and constant, suggesting a change in either her refractive error or the physical characteristics of the lens. A new left contact lens with identical parameters was ordered and dispensed. A recheck 1 month later showed 20/20 visual acuity and no subjective complaints. I discussed the phenomenon of lens warpage with her and reinstructed her in proper handling, cleaning, and storage techniques.

IV. Alternative Management Plan/Summary

Lens warpage can be due to a number of factors: lens material, lens design (especially center thickness), lens fit, corneal toricity, lid structure/tension, and patient handling. Newer RGP materials with a higher permeability constant (Dk) are usually more flexible than the first-generation silicone/acrylate materials. Previous silicone/arcylate RGP wearers who are refitted into newer fluoro-silicone/acrylate materials often need reinstruction in proper handling techniques. Lenses should never be cleaned between the fingers but rather in the palm of the hand, with care taken to exert even and *gentle* pressure. (Fluoro-silicone/acrylate lens surfaces require less mechanical force to remove film and debris.) Lenses should always be stored wet, and the storage well refilled regularly with appropriate conditioning solution. Proper attention must also be given to lens design and fitting. Follow the manufacturer's recommendations for center thickness. Patients with high corneal toricity or repeated warpage problems may require thicker designs than normally advised. Finally, an alignment fitting approach will help minimize lens flexure and thus lens warpage.

Newer fluoro-silicone/acrylate materials can offer significant physiological advantages for many patients and are rapidly becoming the standard of care for RGP wearers. Proper attention to design and fitting will optimize the visual performance and comfort of these new products and ultimately increase patient satisfaction.

Refitting Options for Lens Warpage

Reorder same lens and reinstruct the patient in lens-handling techniques (especially cleaning)

Follow manufacturer's center thickness recommendation and **verify**

Increase center thickness 0.02 mm

Adjust base curve to achieve a more aligned central fit (avoid steep central fit)

Consider toric design if there is over 2.50 D of corneal toricity

Refit into a more rigid material (such as Boston RXD)

C H A P T E R

2

Rigid Lens Care and Compliance

Judith L. Kremer
Edward S. Bennett

One of the most frequent, if not *the* most frequent, reasons for discontinuation of rigid lens wear is either inadequate patient education or poor patient compliance (or both). If a patient leaves the office without feeling proficient at insertion and removal, without having realistic expectations as to wearing time and lens awareness, or without being educated in the proper lens care regimen, failure may result before the practitioner has had an opportunity to correct the error(s). Comprehensive patient education is essential for successful contact lens wear. The purpose of this chapter is to provide essential components of what should be included in the educational process of a new rigid gas-permeable (RGP) lens wearer.

• Case One: Preservative Reaction

I. Subjective Data

A new RGP wearer presented for her 1-week follow-up visit with 30 Dk RGP lenses. Overall, she was very satisfied with her vision and had been experiencing adequate comfort during her efforts to build up wearing time to 10 hours. Her only complaint was that she experienced mild burning and redness every morning upon insertion of her

19

lenses that lasted no more than 10 minutes. She had been using the prescribed solutions, which were preserved with polyaminopropyl biguanide (PAPB).

II. Objective Data

External examination showed a 1+ bulbar conjunctival injection in each eye. Slit-lamp examination revealed a mild diffuse superficial punctate staining of each cornea. All other findings were normal.

III. Assessment/Plan

This patient most likely was suffering from an allergic reaction to the preservative in the solution (Plate 6). She was given a care kit with a solution system containing a different preservative, and care procedures were carefully reviewed. At her 1-month progress check, she denied any burning or redness upon insertion of the lenses and there were no signs of preservative sensitivity upon slit-lamp examination.

IV. Alternative Management Plan/Summary

Fortunately, this patient was compliant in switching solutions as directed. Long-term use of an incompatible preservative can eventually lead to lens intolerance and discontinued wearing of the contact lenses. Preservatives that could have been used in this case are benzalkonium chloride (BAK), thimerosal, chlorhexidine, or benzyl alcohol, since preservative sensitivity is not PAPB specific. Any preservative can produce the symptoms in a given patient. Simply changing to another care system with a different preservative will almost always eliminate this problem.

• Case Two: Inadequate Cleaning

I. Subjective Data

A 17-year-old patient presented for the 1-year progress evaluation on his silicone/acrylate contact lenses. He had noticed decreasing comfort and vision over the preceding 2 months but had not been evaluated in the office for 9 months (he failed to show up for his 6-month progress check). Upon questioning, he gave very brief answers and claimed to be following the prescribed care regimen although he could not recall the names of the solutions he was using.

II. Objective Data

Visual acuity was reduced from a baseline of 20/20 to 20/40 in both eyes. Biomicroscopy revealed grade 2 conjunctival injection in addition to grade 1+ papillary hypertrophy. There was a moderate mucoprotein film, along with numerous scratches, on the surface of both lenses.

Upon further questioning, the patient finally admitted to sporadic use of a daily cleaner (only 1 or 2 times per week) and no use of a wetting/soaking agent. In fact, he was using tap water to wet the lenses before insertion.

III. Assessment/Plan

This patient failed to care for his lenses adequately, resulting in the aforementioned complications. Three steps were taken to allow him to return to successful contact lens wear: First, he was shown photographs of filmy scratched lenses and of giant papillary conjunctivitis (GPC). This helped reinforce for him the potential severity of noncompliance. Second, his lenses were replaced. A low Dk fluoro-silicone/acrylate material was selected. Third, he was reeducated in the proper care procedures for RGP lenses, with emphasis on regular cleaning at night when they are removed and the use of a wetting/soaking agent. He was then asked to sign a custom-designed form that provided specific instructions pertaining to his lens care regimen (Fig. 2-1).

IV. Alternative Management Plan/Summary

If the patient's condition had become moderately severe, it might have been beneficial for him to discontinue contact lens wear for 1 or 2 weeks. However, in this case, simply replacing the lenses produced a dramatic improvement in his physiological status and level of comfort.

In addition to careful documentation of this patient's admitted noncompliance, he should be asked to return for frequent progress evaluations to ensure that he is following the prescribed care regimen. The use of a daily cleaner is important to remove lipids, mucoproteins, and debris. If the surface of the lens is not kept clean, poor surface wettability results. A nonabrasive surfactant cleaner is generally effective, although some patients may require a cleaner that contains abrasive particulate matter. In addition, a weekly enzymatic cleaning is often necessary for more comprehensive protein removal.

For the following reasons it is important that RGP contact lenses be stored in a wetting/soaking solution: to disinfect them, to maintain base curve radius stability, to enhance their wettability, and to minimize surface scratches. The wetting solution also serves numerous functions both before and during insertion including enhancement of surface wettability, disinfection, maintenance of the lens in a hydrated state, and acting as a mechanical buffer between the cornea and contact lens.

• Case Three: Poor Initial Wettability

I. Subjective Data

An experienced RGP lens wearer arrived at the clinic for a spare pair of contact lenses. He mentioned that comfort and vision did not

STATEMENT BY PATIENT   (File Copy)

This is to certify that on _____, 19__ I received instructions in the proper methods of insertion, removal, use and care of my contact lenses. Having proved myself to be competent enough to carry out the above instructions, the contact lenses were given to me. I realize that success with contact lenses cannot be guaranteed and that any refund will be subject to the policy outlined below.

_____   _____
Patient's Signature   Student Clinician's Signature

                                 _____
                                 Instructor's Signature

The solutions prescribed with these _____ contact lenses are:

wetting and rinsing _____

soaking/disinfectant _____

cleaning _____

enzyme cleaner _____

other _____

IN CASE OF EMERGENCY:

Phone: 1. Center for Eye Care, 553-5131 or Contact Lens Clinic, 553-5609
                 during clinic hours.
              2. Student Clinician evenings or weekends (in the case that you
                 require assistance and cannot reach anyone at the clinic)

REFUND POLICY:

Patient discontinued within 60 days from dispensing......50% of total contact lens fees paid is refunded

              After 60 days.. no refund applies

REPLACEMENT POLICY (without savings plan):

    Class A.....................................single $60   pair $105
    Class B.....................................single $75   pair $125
    Class C.....................................single $85   pair $150
    Class D.....................................single $105   pair $185

Your contact lens is Class A B C D and no refund applies after _____

The fitting fee includes lenses, starter kit of solutions and 4 months of contact lens follow-up visits. Follow-up visits are suggested every 6 months after the initial period. The standard fee for a follow-up visit is $20.00. A comprehensive eye examination should be performed every year.

FEE AND COSTS ARE SUBJECT TO PERIODIC REVISIONS

FIGURE 2-1 Patient agreement and education form. (Courtesy Randy McLaughlin.)

appear to be as good as with his old pair although the lens material and all parameters were exactly the same. He also mentioned that occasionally, if he blinked rapidly numerous times, the lenses seemed to provide improved vision and comfort for a few seconds.

II. Objective Data

Upon slit-lamp (biomicroscopic) examination the lenses exhibited poor initial wettability; the tear break-up time (B.U.T.) over the lenses was only 3 seconds despite the fact that the lenses were soaked in wetting solution for 24 hours before being dispensed. In addition, wetting solution was rubbed into the surface of the lenses immediately before insertion.

III. Assessment/Plan

The contact lenses were cleaned with a laboratory cleaner, wetting solution was applied, and the lenses were reinserted. The patient noticed improved comfort and visual acuity, and slit-lamp examination of the lenses revealed significantly improved surface wettability. The tear B.U.T. over the lenses was now 10 seconds.

IV. Alternative Management Plan/Summary

The most likely cause for poor initial wettability is residual pitch polish from the laboratory on the surface of the lens. This is removed most efficiently by a laboratory cleaner, such as Fluoro-Solve or Boston Laboratory Cleaner, although in many cases the problem can be eliminated simply by presoaking the lenses overnight in the recommended soaking solution. If the laboratory cleaner is unsuccessful in providing good surface wettability, a light surface polish is often successful. Laboratories experienced in the manufacturing of RGP contact lenses should routinely remove any residual pitch polish. If the polish routinely becomes an observable problem, the laboratory should be contacted and the services of a different laboratory considered.

> **CLINICAL PEARL**
>
> *The most likely cause for poor initial wettability is residual pitch polish from the laboratory on the surface of the lens. This is removed most efficiently by a laboratory cleaner, such as Fluoro-Solve or Boston Laboratory Cleaner, although in many cases the problem can be eliminated simply by presoaking the lenses overnight in the recommended soaking solution.*

• Case Four: Warpage

I. Subjective Data

A former polymethyl methacrylate (PMMA) lens–wearing patient was refitted into a pair of extended-wear RGP contact lenses and asked to return for a follow-up examination in 1 week. He failed to show up for the exam but did return 6 months later complaining of blurry vision. Visual acuity was 20/30+2 OD, 20/25−3 OS.

II. Objective Data

The overrefraction was −0.25 − 0.75 × 175 OD and +0.25 − 1.00 × 005 OS. The base curve radii, initially 7.75 mm OU, were now verified as 7.70 × 7.81 mm OD and 7.68 × 7.80 mm OS. Both lenses were significantly warped. Upon being asked to demonstrate his cleaning technique, the patient rubbed the lens between his thumb and index finger.

III. Assessment/Plan

Excessive pressure on the contact lenses during cleaning caused them to become warped. The patient was ordered a new pair (again extended-wear) and was thoroughly educated in the correct method of cleaning RGP lenses. He was told to use very light pressure and to clean them in the palm of his hand with a back-and-forth rather than circular motion. In addition, the importance of follow-up care was explained and the patient was encouraged to return to the office every 3 months (as directed for all extended-wear patients).

IV. Alternative Management Plan/Summary

Former PMMA wearers often have developed habits that are contraindicated in RGP wear. Warpage has been shown[4] to be a much greater problem for them than for other patients. When dealing with former PMMA wearers, it is extremely important to emphasize comprehensive patient education. This should assist in minimizing problems such as the case described here. Other areas to address include the importance of soaking the lenses overnight in the prescribed wetting/soaking solution, the careful handling of lenses to prevent scratches, and the avoidance of using saliva, toothpaste, dishwashing detergent, liquid soap, etc. on lenses for cleaning and/or wetting.

If this patient continues to warp his lenses regularly, it may become necessary to prescribe a lower-Dk material for him, and to limit him to daily wear only. In fact, recommending this initially might have eliminated the warpage problem. Likewise, a "hands-off" system such as the Hydra-Mat (PBH) or the De Stat 3/Stay-Wet 3 regimen (Sherman Pharmaceuticals) can be prescribed.

• Case Five: "Left Lens Syndrome"

I. Subjective Data

A new patient with a 4-year history of RGP contact lens wear visited our clinic for the purpose of a refit. She commented that both comfort and vision with her 2-year-old contact lenses had been better for the first few months of wear than for the past year. She had been wearing them only on an occasional basis because they were too uncomfortable for more than 6 hours at a stretch. Symptoms included dryness, redness and itchiness, which were slightly worse in the left eye than the right. She claimed to clean the lenses after wearing them but admitted that she had failed to perform this step a few times. Enzymatic cleaning was not part of her lens care regimen.

II. Objective Data

Upon slit-lamp (biomicroscopic) examination the lenses centered well and showed an "on K" fitting relationship with the cornea. There was excessive movement with the blink. Both lenses exhibited a significant mucoprotein film, with the left lens being more coated than the right. There was also poor surface wettability. The patient had grade 1+ injection of the bulbar conjunctiva in the right eye, grade 2 in the left. A papillary reaction of her palpebral conjunctiva showed a slight difference between the eyes: grade 2 OD and grade 2+ OS. Both corneas had a very mild diffuse superficial punctate keratitis.

III. Assessment/Plan

All the signs and symptoms in this case could be attributed to both sporadic cleaning and an absence of enzymatic cleaning, which resulted in filmy lenses causing poor long-term surface wettability (Plate 7). A papillary reaction followed, leading to excessive contact lens movement. In combination, these problems produced redness, a diffuse superficial punctate keratitis, and the general decreased comfort and vision experienced by the patient. The fact that her left eye showed more severe signs could be attributed to the so-called "left lens syndrome." To alleviate these problems, new lenses were ordered and the patient was thoroughly educated in proper lens cleaning techniques. An enzymatic cleaner was prescribed for weekly use. Her wearing time was maintained under 8 hours a day initially, allowing the ocular health to return to normal. In addition, rewetting drops were prescribed, to be used at least bid.

IV. Alternative Management Plan/Summary

The "left lens syndrome" pertains to the problem of patients who clean their right lens first and more thoroughly than the left, eventually causing the left lens to become more deposit-bound and problematical (including papillary hypertrophy, reduced wearing time, etc.) than the right.[2] Often simply bringing this potential problem to the attention of the patient will prevent its occurrence. Enzymatic cleaning should be prescribed not only for patients who have exhibited deposit problems but also for borderline dry-eye patients and extended-wear patients. Rewetting drops are also beneficial for many patients; they are designed to perform the following functions[5]: (1) rewet the lens surface, (2) stabilize the tear film, (3) rinse away trapped debris, and (4) break up loosely attached deposits. Patient education in these topics at the dispensing visit will certainly help alleviate many potential problems.

CLINICAL PEARL

The "left lens syndrome" pertains to the problem of patients who clean their right lens first and more thoroughly than the left, eventually causing the left lens to become more deposit bound and problematical (including papillary hypertrophy, reduced wearing time, etc.) than the right.[2] Often simply bringing this potential problem to the attention of the patient will prevent its occurrence.

• Case 6: Change in Lens Power

I. Subjective Data

A 38-year-old man presented with a chief complaint of blurry vision, especially at near, with his 2-year-old low-Dk-fluoro-silicone/acrylate contact lenses. He claimed that he was very good about using his prescribed daily cleaner and wetting/soaking agent (Boston Cleaner and Boston Conditioner). He admitted to cleaning the lenses between his index finger and thumb.

II. Objective Data

Distance visual acuities were 20/20-2 OD and 20/20 OS. Near visual acuities were decreased to 20/25 in each eye. Slit-lamp examination showed the lenses to be well centered, with adequate movement, and a slightly "flatter than K" fitting relationship with the cornea. The lenses were minimally filmy and had a few scratches. The anterior segment of each eye was clear and healthy. The overrefraction resulted in +1.00 DS OU and visual acuity equal to 20/15-2 OD and 20/15-1 OS. Verification of the lenses revealed an increase in minus power OU of −1.00 DS. In addition, the center thickness of each lens had decreased 0.05 mm. The lenses were not warped.

III. Assessment/Plan

A significant increase in minus power had resulted from the long-term use of an abrasive surfactant cleaner in combination with a digital technique to clean the lenses. The patient was educated in the proper method of cleaning RGP contact lenses: in the palm, with a back-and-forth motion, and using gentle pressure. New contact lenses were ordered. It was interesting to note that this patient had noticed the increased power at near since he was approaching presbyopia.

CLINICAL PEARL

A significant increase in minus power had resulted from the long-term use of an abrasive surfactant cleaner in combination with a digital technique to clean the lenses. The patient was educated in the proper method of cleaning RGP contact lenses: in the palm, with a back-and-forth motion, and using gentle pressure.

IV. Alternative Management Plan/Summary

It has been shown that abrasive surfactant cleaners can cause an increase in minus power.[3] If this patient had continued to add minus power to his lenses, despite meticulous education, it might have become necessary for him to clean his lenses using a hands-off approach as described in Case Four. Other options would have been to switch to a nonabrasive cleaner, or even a surfactant soaking cleaner. Also, if this patient had continued to have trouble at near with the new contact lenses, perhaps he would have benefited from a reading correction.

• Case Seven: Improper Use of Solution

I. Subjective Data

A long-time RGP lens wearer called the office for an emergency work-in appointment. He had experienced a burning sensation and his eyes had become red and painful upon insertion of his contact lenses that morning. However, his symptoms had diminished by the time he called the office, 3 hours later. He had been examined the day before and was asymptomatic at that time. He mentioned that he had been given a sample kit of some new solutions and tried these for the first time last night. The new system included one solution with combination wetting/rewetting capabilities and one with cleaning/disinfection capabilities. His previous regimen had a soaking agent that was separate from the cleaner.

II. Objective Data

The bulbar conjunctiva of both eyes exhibited 2+ injection, and the corneas showed a moderate diffuse superficial punctate keratitis. There was a grade 1 corneal edema. Visual acuity was slightly decreased to 20/25 OU.

III. Assessment/Plan

This patient had inadvertently used his cleaning agent, which also serves as a soaking agent, to wet the lens for insertion. He was advised to use preservative-free rewetting drops qh for the remainder of the day and to resume contact lens wear the following day if symptoms were alleviated. The differences between the two solutions were explained thoroughly to him and he was scheduled to return in 6 months for a follow-up examination.

IV. Alternative Management Plan/Summary

This case demonstrates the importance of thoroughly explaining each stage of RGP lens care. A sample solution kit should not be provided to patients unless they are educated as to how to use it. This is not usually a problem with RGP lens solutions since most employ the same type of solutions and procedures. However, it is important to make sure that patients are aware that not all systems are used identically. This situation could have been avoided altogether if the patient had been educated correctly.

• Case Eight: Poor Hygiene

I. Subjective Data

A patient presented for his 6-month check on new RGP contact lenses. His only complaint was that his lower eyelids itched and he had a large amount of mucus in both eyes throughout the day.

II. Objective Data

The external examination revealed somewhat poor hygiene. The patient appeared to have oily skin and hair and had dirt under his fingernails. When asked about his lens care regimen, he pulled his solutions out of a bag he had brought to the appointment. The contact lens case was heavily contaminated, as were the bottles of solutions. He admitted to "topping off" his disinfecting solution, or adding a small amount to top off what was already in the case instead of replacing the solution every night. Biomicroscopy revealed grade 1+ injection, scales along the eyelash follicles, and mild punctate staining of the inferior third of the cornea. Visual acuity was 20/20 OU.

III. Assessment/Plan

This patient had developed chronic blepharitis and bacterial conjunctivitis as a result of poor contact lens hygiene. The first step taken to educate him was to discard his old case and solutions and to warn him against the risks of sight-threatening complications that can result from "topping off" solutions (Plate 8). For the blepharitis and conjunctivitis, he was prescribed a mild antibiotic drop to be used qid for 10 days. In addition, it was recommended that he use lid scrubs and cool compresses bid. He was also instructed to wash his hands thoroughly before handling the lenses and to discontinue contact lens wear for 2 days while correctly cleaning and disinfecting the lenses every day.

IV. Alternative Management Plan/Summary

Proper lens hygiene should be emphasized during the contact lens educational process. If not carefully educated, many patients will learn poor habits. This case illustrates the importance of careful questioning at follow-up visits about the patient's RGP lens care routine. If he had continued to show poor hygiene, it might eventually have become necessary to discontinue him from contact lens wear altogether. In addition, it would have been a good idea to have him sign a document explaining that he understood the contact lens care regimen and agreed to adhere to it.

• Case Nine: Inadequate Education

I. Subjective Data

A new patient was fitted with daily wear RGP contact lenses. She received her lenses on the same day as her examination and was given very little instruction or education by her doctor. The staff mistakenly assumed that she was familiar with handling and caring for RGP contact lenses, so she was not scheduled for a patient education class. She was asked to return in 2 weeks for a follow-up examination. When she arrived for this appointment, she was very discouraged and her contact lenses were in the case. She had been noticing increased photophobia and redness when she wore them and was afraid that they might be harming her eyes. She had not worn the lenses since the day after her initial examination.

II. Objective Data

This patient was so discouraged that she initially wanted a full refund. However, with persuasion, she eventually allowed the contact lenses to be placed on her eyes for evaluation. The lens/cornea fitting relationship was excellent and provided her with 20/20 visual acuity in each eye.

III. Assessment/Plan

This patient did not receive proper education about what to expect from her RGP contact lenses. She had felt rushed through the examination and was about to become an "RGP failure." Fortunately, she became encouraged when the doctor explained that the lens fit was perfect and that it was normal to feel uncertain about handling and caring for new lenses. She then proceeded to attend the usual contact lens education class provided for all new lens wearers (this had been overlooked initially). Normal symptoms of RGP adaptation (tearing, minor irritation, intermittent blurry vision, light sensitivity, and mild redness) and abnormal ones (sudden pain, severe redness, and prolonged blur) were reviewed. She was told to build her wearing time up slowly—beginning with 4 hours of wear and increasing by 2 hours every other day—and to return for a progress examination in 1 week. She left the office feeling confident and comfortable with her lenses.

IV. Alternative Management Plan/Summary

The office should have been more prepared for this patient. Because of an oversight, she could easily have discontinued lens wear altogether. There are many points to be learned from this case: First, proper patient education is critical to success. Patients need to know exactly what to expect. Second, it is important to reexamine the patient within 1 week instead of 2. The initial progress examination is primarily for subjective rather than objective purposes; it allows the practitioner to question the patient about lens care while clearing up any misunderstandings. In addition, it can be beneficial for a member of the staff to call all new contact lens wearers within 2 or 3 days to address any potential difficulties.

CLINICAL PEARL

The initial progress examination is primarily for subjective rather than objective purposes; it allows the practitioner to question the patient about lens care while clearing up any misunderstandings.

• Case Ten: Difficulty with Insertion and Removal

I. Subjective Data

A 66-year-old man was fitted with RGP contact lenses for aphakia. He returned for his 1-week progress evaluation feeling frustrated with handling the lenses. He mentioned that his wife had to insert and remove the lenses for him, since he could not seem to master the procedure himself. He said he had been able to insert and remove the lenses once before he took them home but then had failed to remember the technique after he left the office.

II. Objective Data

The patient was asked to demonstrate his technique for the optometric technician. He seemed to be having the most trouble just relaxing enough to properly handle the lenses.

III. Assessment/Plan

The technician provided specific instructions and hints to help him with handling the lenses. She followed a four-step education process—written instructions, verbal reinforcement, video, and reeducation. A written instruction manual was given to the patient. This type of manual should be comprehensive yet easily followed and should provide the information listed in the box. The use of a video is especially beneficial when the patient is uncertain about technique, because it can be sent home for reviewing. Patient reeducation at follow-up visits is also invaluable. It has been shown[6] that patients are more compliant when instructions are reinforced at follow-up.

 Important Information for the RGP Lens Patient Education Manual

1. What is an RGP lens?
2. RGP benefits?
3. Insertion, removal, and decentration (with diagrams and photographs if possible)
4. How to properly clean an RGP lens
5. Normal and abnormal adaptation symptoms
6. Causes of reduced wear (e.g., colds, hay fever, medications)
7. Importance of adhering to prescribed wearing schedule
8. Importance of using the recommended care regimen (not saliva or nonrecommended brands); alternative acceptable solutions
9. How to minimize loss and surface damage
10. Benefits of a spare pair of lenses and spectacles
11. Use with cosmetics
12. Swimming
13. Caring for the lens case
14. Visit schedule
15. Fee and refund policy
16. Service agreement
17. Office telephone and emergency number

IV. Alternative Management Plan/Summary

Most patients have a difficult time when first confronted with the insertion and removal of RGP contact lenses. A good rule-of-thumb to follow when dispensing lenses to first-time wearers is to make sure they can demonstrate their ability to insert and remove the lenses before taking them home.

CLINICAL PEARL

A good rule-of-thumb to follow when dispensing lenses to first-time wearers is to make sure they can demonstrate their ability to insert and remove the lenses before taking them home.

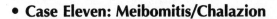

• Case Eleven: Meibomitis/Chalazion

I. Subjective Data

A 53-year-old RGP wearer presented to the office complaining of a "bump" on her left lower lid for the past 5 days. She was not experiencing any pain but was discouraged by the appearance of the bump. She obviously was concerned about her appearance, because she wore a heavy amount of makeup.

II. Objective Data

Upon slit-lamp examination, it was found that she had a 2 mm chalazion on her lower lid. Examination of the lid margins revealed meibomian gland plugs, due to her wearing of eyeliner, along the inner lid margin. Her tear film was very oily, and her contact lenses were moderately coated.

III. Assessment/Plan

This patient was prescribed warm compresses and lid scrubs tid to alleviate the meibomitis and chalazion. She was educated on the use of cosmetics in conjunction with contact lenses. In addition, her lenses were cleaned with a laboratory cleaner and polished.

IV. Alternative Management Plan/Summary

If this patient had continued to have cosmetic-related contact lens complications, it might have become necessary for her to discontinue lens wear until the condition cleared. Replacement of her contact lenses could have temporarily improved the condition, but to find a long-term solution it would have been necessary to change her habits.

Every contact lens patient should be thoroughly educated in the proper use of cosmetics. Because many cosmetics contain ingredients such as preservatives, pigments, oils, and solvents, subjective discomfort and eye infection can result from their use.[1] Lenses should be inserted before cosmetics are applied. Nylon or rayon fibers from "lash-building" mascara can flake off into the tear film, become trapped behind the lens, and cause a corneal abrasion. Bacterial contamination of cosmetics can also be a problem. A patient may transfer bacteria from her lashes to the mascara wand and then into the mascara tube, where they colonize.

There are numerous cosmetic products on the market that are recommended for contact lens patients. They are water soluble and contain little or no fragrances, fillers, or oils. It is also important for patients to thoroughly wash their hands of any residual cosmetic product before handling the lenses. Many optically compatible soaps are available that contain no oils, perfumes, or dyes. It is a good idea to recommend these to all contact lens patients.

• Case Twelve: Changing Care Regimen Due to Cost

I. Subjective Data

An RGP patient presented with the chief complaint of redness, itching, and burning that had begun immediately after using her new solutions. Upon questioning, she admitted to having purchased some generic solutions because they were less expensive. She said that she could not recall the names of the solutions that had been originally prescribed.

II. Objective Data

Biomicroscopic examination revealed the same clinical signs as were observed in Case One. This patient had a preservative-induced solution reaction from using inappropriate solutions.

III. Assessment/Plan

Patient reeducation was important in this case. Once again, she was provided with a form listing the recommended solutions. In addition, she was given full-size bottles of her cleaning and wetting/soaking solutions so she would be more likely to recognize them in the store. She was also prescribed preservative-free rewetting drops to be used q2h for the remainder of the day.

IV. Alternative Management Plan/Summary

The large number of currently available contact lens care products makes patient compliance challenging. Patients frequently have a difficult time remembering which solutions they have been told to use. Price may be another reason for solution switching; often patients will buy a solution just because it is less expensive. Solution switching can be minimized by:

1. Thoroughly educating the patient about which solutions and alternative solutions can be used.
2. Emphasizing *why* certain solutions are recommended. This will help discourage price shopping.
3. At follow-up examinations, asking the patient which solutions he or she has been using. Asking open questions will obtain honest answers.
4. Providing a large supply of solutions to every patient initially.
5. Selling solutions in the office at a low price.

CLINICAL PEARL

Solution switching can be minimized by:
1. *Thoroughly educating the patient about which solutions and alternative solutions can be used.*
2. *Emphasizing why certain solutions are recommended. This will help discourage price shopping.*
3. *At follow-up examinations, asking the patient which solutions he or she has been using. Asking open questions will obtain honest answers.*
4. *Providing a large supply of solutions to every patient initially.*
5. *Selling solutions in the office at a low price.*

Summary

As these cases demonstrate, comprehensive patient education is essential for success. If contact lenses are to become increasingly popular as a corrective option, patient goodwill is vital. Patient goodwill can be achieved through a positive experience with lens wear. This positive experience is often obtained from confidence achieved at the patient education visit.

Bibliography

1 Baldwin JS: Cosmetics: too long concealed as culprit in eye problems, *Contact Lens Forum* 11:38, 1986.

2 Bennett ES, Grohe RM, Snyder C: Lens care and patient education. In Bennett ES, Weissman BA: *Clinical contact lens practice,* Philadelphia, 1993, JB Lippincott, pp 25-1 to 25-11.

3 Carrell BA, Bennett ES, Henry VA, Grohe RM: The effect of rigid gas permeable lens cleaners on lens parameter stability, *J Am Optom Assoc* 63:193, 1992.

4 Henry VA, Bennett ES, Forrest J: Clinical investigation of the Paraperm EW rigid gas-permeable contact lens, *Am J Optom Physiol Opt* 64:313, 1987.

5 Sibley MJ, Barr JT, et al: Lubricating and rewetting solutions: a roundtable discussion, *Contact Lens Spectrum* 4:41, 1989.

6 Wilson LA, Sawant AD, Simmons RB, et al: Microbial contamination of contact lens storage cases and solutions, *Am J Ophthalmol* 110:193-198, 1990.

3

Hydrogel Lens Fitting, Evaluation, and Problem Solving

Vinita Allee Henry
William G. Bachman

The importance of carefully evaluating and monitoring soft lens–wearing patients can hardly be overemphasized. It is not uncommon for complications to result simply because the patient was monitored insufficiently and the fitting relationship and/or lens material needed to be changed. This chapter addresses several cases pertaining to soft contact lens design, fitting, and problem solving.

• Case One: Good Soft Lens Candidate

I. Subjective Data

A mother brought her 15-year-old son to our clinic to be fitted with contact lenses. He had never worn them before. She said he was very responsible, and he appeared to be motivated to care for the lenses. He played soccer and basketball at school.

II. Objective Data

Manifest refraction

OD: −2.00 DS (20/20)
OS: −1.50 DS (20/20)

Keratometry

OD: 43.00 @ 180; 43.25 @ 090 (smooth mires)
OS: 43.00 @ 180; 43.25 @ 090 (smooth mires)

Biomicroscopy

Biomicroscopy revealed healthy normal corneas and a tear break-up time (B.U.T.) of 12 seconds OU.

III. Assessment/Plan

This patient was considered to be an excellent candidate for hydrogel lenses because of his spherical refraction and healthy ocular findings and his athletic lifestyle. He was fitted with a medium–center thickness (approximately 0.06 mm) low–water content lens with a visibility tint. The final lenses ordered were 8.6 mm base curve radius OU with powers equal to the refraction, OD −2.00 D and OS −1.50 D.

IV. Alternative Management Plan/Summary

Acceptable center thicknesses would be any of the daily-wear lenses that are 0.06 mm or thicker. First-time wearers often have difficulty handling hydrogel lenses, especially in powers under −2.50 D. It is easy for the edges of a lens to stick together or for the patient to tear an ultrathin lens. In addition, ultrathin lenses may be more difficult to insert because of folding or adhering to the finger. For these reasons the medium- to standard-thickness lenses handle best. Some examples of lenses that fall into this category are the Optima 38, the Cibasoft and Ciba STD, and the CSI. In addition, first-time wearers will benefit from tinted lenses so they can see them out of the eye. In this case the patient was fitted with visibility tinted lenses, but even an enhancing or opaque-tinted lens would be acceptable if the patient desires a tint.

• Case Two: Flat-Fitting Lens

Part One: Edge Standoff

I. Subjective Data

A 14-year-old girl came to our clinic interested in soft lens wear. She was becoming progressively myopic, and cosmesis with spectacles was a strong motivating factor. She did not have any allergies and was not taking any medications.

II. Objective Data

Manifest refraction

OD: −4.25 − 0.25 × 175 (20/15)
OS: −3.75 − 0.25 × 180 (20/20 +2)

Keratometry

OD: 43.75 @ 180; 44.25 @ 090
OS: 44.00 @ 180; 44.50 @ 090

Biomicroscopy

She showed no evidence of ocular compromise at biomicroscopic examination. The tear film quality was normal, the lids were satin in appearance, and no corneal staining was present.

Diagnostic lenses

Because the patient did not have a preference for daily or extended wear, she was fitted into a planned-replacement regimen with the B & L Medalist. Her initial diagnostic lenses were

		BCR	OAD	Power
OD:	Medalist	8.7 mm	14.0 mm	−4.00 D
OS:	Medalist	8.7 mm	14.0 mm	−3.75 D

Biomicroscopy with contact lenses

Both contact lenses exhibited good centration, with about 1 mm of movement after the blink. However, the patient indicated that they felt uncomfortable. Upon further evaluation, both lenses were found to have slight edge standoff inferonasally. When the patient looked down, they tended to decenter superotemporally. They were then removed to verify that they had not become inverted on the eye.

III. Assessment/Plan

It was evident that edge standoff was compromising the fitting relationship. This inferior or inferolateral curling of the lens edge is caused by selecting too flat a base curve radius. It is recommended to always have the patient look downward to ensure that the lens is tucking underneath the lower lid. Although this problem is predictable if a flat base curve radius lens is selected on a steeper than average corneal curvature (e.g., a 9.0 mm BCR on a 46.00 DS cornea), it can also result unpredictably as in this case. Often it is due to an unusual corneal topography not consistent with the keratometry values. In this case the following lenses were fitted:

		BCR	OAD	Power	Overrefraction
OD:	Medalist	8.4 mm	14.0 mm	−4.25 D	Plano (20/20)
OS:	Medalist	8.4 mm	14.0 mm	−3.75 D	Plano (20/20)

CLINICAL PEARL

This inferior or inferolateral curling of the lens edge is caused by selecting too flat a base curve radius. It is recommended to always have the patient look downward to ensure that the lens is tucking underneath the lower lid.

Biomicroscopy with contact lenses

Good centration and lens movement were present OU. Upon downward gaze, both lenses tucked underneath the lower lid. There was no evidence of edge standoff. It was decided to provide the patient with these lenses.

Part Two: Inferior Decentration

I. Subjective Data

A 16-year-old boy with progressive myopia who had worn spectacles since he was 12 wanted contact lenses because he disliked glasses, especially when participating in sports. He played for his high school basketball and golf teams. He had had no allergies and was not currently taking any medications. He did appear to exhibit a greater than average anxiety during lid eversion and applanation tonometry, however.

II. Objective Data

Manifest refraction

OD: $-2.75 -0.25 \times 170$ (20/20 +1)
OS: -2.50 DS   (20/15)

Keratometry

OD: 43.25 @ 180; 43.75 @ 090 (smooth mires)
OS: 43.50 DS (smooth mires)

Biomicroscopy

He showed no evidence of ocular compromise at biomicroscopic examination. The tear film quality was normal, his lids were satin in appearance, and no corneal staining was present.

    Based on the patient's desire for soft lenses, his participation in athletics (especially basketball), his apprehension about something touching his eyes, and his spherical refractive error—a spherical hydrogel was the contact lens of choice. The CSI lens was selected because of its deposit resistance.

Diagnostic lenses

		BCR	OAD	Power
OD:	CSI	8.6 mm	13.8 mm	-2.75 D
OS:	CSI	8.6 mm	13.8 mm	-2.50 D

The lenses exhibited good centration with 1 mm of movement on straight-ahead gaze. However, on upward gaze they quickly decentered inferiorly onto the sclera.

III. Assessment/Plan

The lenses selected for this patient should, in theory, position well on his corneas. However, both decentered upon upward gaze. As in Part

One of this case, keratometry readings are not always predictive of which lenses will be successful on a given patient. He was refitted into the following steeper base curve radii:

		BCR	OAD	Power
OD:	CSI	8.3 mm	13.8 mm	−2.75 D
OS:	CSI	8.3 mm	13.8 mm	−2.50 D

Biomicroscopy with contact lenses

Both contact lenses were positioned similarly to the 8.6 mm base curve radius lenses. However, on upward gaze they did not shift inferiorly. The patient was given these lenses.

It is important to evaluate lenses in the upward as well as straight-ahead gaze. When a lens shifts inferiorly, it is often due to an unusual corneal topography; and, although not always successful, the selection of a steeper base curve radius may solve the problem.

CLINICAL PEARL

It is therefore important to evaluate the lenses in upward as well as straight-ahead gaze. When the lens shifts inferiorly, it is often due to an unusual corneal topography; and, although not always successful, selecting a steeper base curve radius may solve the problem.

IV. Alternative Management Plan/Summary

In both these cases the initial diagnostic lenses were too flat, as evidenced by edge standoff or inferior decentration. However, in neither case would the keratometry readings alone have predicted the need for a steeper base curve radius. Individual variations in corneal topography often necessitate selecting a lens that is either flatter or steeper than predicted. Selecting a steeper base curve radius was successful in both cases. Other management options to consider if a base curve radius change does not have an effect would include a thinner lens (e.g., CSI-T) or a larger-diameter lens (e.g., 14.5 mm). Obviously, it is important to apply diagnostic lenses and never assume that a certain base curve–radius lens is going to be successful without a comprehensive biomicroscopic evaluation of the lens in primary, upward, and downward gazes.

• Case Three: Ocular Trauma

I. Subjective Data

A 15-year-old boy reported to our clinic with the desire for a prosthetic soft lens. He had experienced ocular trauma to his right eye 6 months earlier resulting in aphakia with a large and distorted pupil.

He was displeased with the cosmetic appearance of this eye and was currently wearing a spectacle correction that included a balance lens for it.

II. Objective Data

Manifest refraction

OD: +14.00 − 0.75 × 078 (20/30)
OS: −1.00 DS (20/20 +2)

Keratometry

OD: 40.75 @ 075; 42.25 @ 165 (mires distorted)
OS: 42.25 @ 180; 42.50 @ 090 (smooth mires)

Biomicroscopy

The right cornea showed an extensive region of midperipheral and peripheral corneal scarring from 2 to 6 o'clock. Otherwise, the cornea, lids, and tear film of each eye were normal. The left eye had a blue iris.

III. Assessment/Plan

The patient was fitted with sapphire blue Durasoft opaque lenses OU. For the right eye a special prosthetic lens was prescribed that provided a good match with the original eye color. The patient was quite satisfied with the artificial iris and smaller regular pupil on the prosthetic lens. Cosmesis was excellent.

IV. Alternative Management Plan/Summary

There are other companies that provide tinted lenses for cosmesis due to ocular trauma. They will also provide a black pupil for a nonseeing eye if desired. At least three companies offer this type of lens: Narcissus Contact Lens (1-415-992-8924 or 9224), PBH CTL-M (1-800-854-6613 or, in California, 1-800-532-3778), and Wesley-Jessen Prosthetic Lens Program (1-800-735-2020). It is always important to consider the individual needs of the patient. This is a good example of how a patient's life can be changed by simply making the effort to determine what prosthetic lenses are available.

• Case Four: Myopic Refractive Change

I. Subjective Data

A 23-year-old patient originally visited our clinic to be fitted with lenses she could wear daily and occasionally overnight. She was fitted with a low–water content thin flexible-wear lens. One year later she is quite successfully wearing these lenses, with only occasional extended wear. At that time she was planning a 2-week trip to Europe and wanted to have extended-wear lenses for the trip. Since she had experienced no problems with short-term extended wear, she decided to wear the lenses with a 10 days on, 1 night off regimen. Three months later she visits the clinic complaining that street signs are difficult to read while driving.

II. Objective Data

Visual acuity with contact lenses

		Overrefraction
OD:	20/40 +2	−1.00 DS 20/20 +1
OS:	20/30 +1	−0.75 DS 20/20 +2

Manifest refraction

OD: −5.00 DS (20/20 −1)
OS: −5.50 − 0.25 × 175 (20/20)

Keratometry

OD: 44.12 @ 180; 44.25 @ 090 (smooth mires)
OS: 44.00 @ 180; 44.25 @ 090 (smooth mires)

Biomicroscopy

Although corneal striae were not observed, the cornea appeared to be slightly hazy or edematous.

It should be mentioned that the patient had increased myopia from a baseline manifest refraction equal to −4.25 DS in the right eye and −4.75 DS in the left. The keratometry readings in both eyes had also steepened approximately 0.50 D from baseline.

III. Assessment/Plan

From a corneal physiological standpoint, some patients cannot tolerate extended-wear. This woman was experiencing the so-called "myopic creep" phenomenon resulting from lens overwear—a progressive increase in myopia that results from chronic corneal hypoxia and often occurs in extended wear. She had never been monitored while wearing the lenses on an extended-wear basis since this was a deviation from her original flexible-wear schedule. In addition, the maximum extended-wear schedule should be 7 days with an overnight break, not 10 days to 2 weeks. Treatment for "myopic creep" in this case was to reduce lens wear to a 12-hour maximum schedule until the keratometry readings and subjective refraction returned to baseline values.

After 3 months of monitoring, her manifest refraction stabilized at

OD: −4.50 DS (20/20 +2)
OS: −5.00 − 0.25 × 180 (20/20)

She was then advised that any overnight wear should be only limited in nature, and she agreed based on the complications she had experienced in the past. She was told that monitoring would occur every 3 months and to contact the clinic if she had any problems.

IV. Alternative Management Plan/Summary

It is unlikely, but if she wished to have full-time extended-wear lenses, she might be refitted into a lens that transmitted more oxygen by increasing the water content (e.g., a 55% water content 0.05 mm center thickness lens). She would then require frequent monitoring, however, to prevent the continued increase of corneal hypoxia. If this was not successful, a refit into RGP extended-wear lenses might provide her with the wearing schedule she desired.

In addition, patient compliance with the recommended wearing schedule must not be underestimated. Patients need to be told at the initial fitting visit about the potential problems of chronic hypoxia. The use of a video (e.g., CLMA/RGPLI Video Library) or photographs is extremely beneficial for this purpose. Myopic creep is often reversible but, if the oxygen supply to the cornea is not increased, may become permanent. In this case the myopia never did return to baseline values.

• Case Five: Borderline Dry Eye

I. Subjective Data

A 21-year-old woman was fitted with lenses 3 months before this visit. Although she enjoyed wearing hydrogel contact lenses, she complained that her eyes felt dry. Lately, she had been experiencing a reduction in wearing time (from 16 to 10 hours) because of the dryness. She did not suffer from any allergies, was not currently taking any medications, and denied being pregnant.

II. Objective Data

Visual acuity with hydrogel lenses

OD: 20/20
OS: 20/20

Manifest refraction

OD: −6.00 DS (20/20)
OS: −5.75 − 0.50 × 010 (20/15-2)

Biomicroscopy

Slit-lamp biomicroscopy revealed a tear break-up time (B.U.T.) of 7 seconds OD and 6 seconds OS. Diffuse corneal staining was present OU.

Current contact lens specifications

	Power	CT
55% water	−5.75 D	0.06 mm

Biomicroscopy with hydrogel lenses

Both lenses showed a mild mucoprotein surface deposition. In addition, less than 0.5 mm of lens movement was present after the blink in straight-ahead gaze compared to 1 mm of movement OU at baseline.

III. Assessment/Plan

This patient was experiencing dry eye symptoms and clinical signs. These problems could have resulted from dehydration of a thin high–water content lens and caused a reduction in both lens movement and oxygen transmission. She was refitted into a low–water content (38%) thicker (0.10 mm) Ciba STD hydrogel lens. Contact lenses with higher water content will further dehydrate an already dry eye. Thick lenses are optimal for dry eyes because the lens mass is increased, thus increasing lens movement and minimizing adherence. By refitting this patient into a low–water content thick hydrogel lens, the dry-eye symptoms were eliminated and wearing time increased.

CLINICAL PEARL

By refitting this patient into a low–water content thick hydrogel lens, the dry-eye symptoms were eliminated and wearing time increased.

IV. Alternative Management Plan/Summary

Several options are possible for the borderline dry eye patient. Certainly a disposable lens would have been selected for daily wear, although in this case the preferable option was a B & L Seequence II because of its low water content. In addition, a non-HEMA (hydroxyethyl methacrylate) hydrogel lens material such as the CSI might have been successful. Of course, rigid gas-permeable (RGP) lenses are beneficial in some dry eye cases because of their enhanced surface wettability. Although this patient continued to be successful, if symptoms had persisted supplemental use of rewetting drops would have been indicated. Likewise, it might have become necessary to limit her wearing time. She could also have removed her lenses during the middle of the wearing schedule for a few minutes to rehydrate and soak them in saline before reinserting. If all else failed punctal occlusion might have been considered. Another factor that could have influenced this patient's dry eye symptoms is her work environment (such as vents that circulate air toward the eyes or prolonged computer use). This should always be investigated, because there may be a simple solution to the dry eye symptoms.

In summary: Borderline dry-eye patients desiring contact lens wear are numerous. They should be questioned about any medications, possible pregnancy, their work environment, and any symptoms of dryness. Evaluation of tear film quality and corneal integrity is also essential. The available solutions are many. In this particular case, switching to a lower–water content thicker lens reduced the effects of dehydration and resulted in a successful and satisfied contact lens wearer.

• Case Six: Torn Lens

I. Subjective Data

A 32-year-old woman who was a new (about a 1 month) daily-wear hydrogel contact lens patient brought in a torn lens (OS) that was replaced by our technician. She returned to the office with the complaint that vision in her right eye was blurred and uncomfortable and the eye felt "scratchy." These symptoms had begun upon lens insertion that morning.

II. Objective Data

Visual acuity with contact lenses

OD: 20/20 +2
OS: 20/20 +1

Manifest refraction

OD: −1.25 − 0.25 × 175 (20/15 −1)
OS: −1.50 DS (20/15 −2)

Biomicroscopy

Fluorescein application resulted in a midperipheral arcuate staining pattern on the right cornea. The left cornea is clear.

Current contact lens specifications

		BCR	OAD	Power	CT
OU:	CSI-T	8.6 mm	13.8 mm	−1.50 D	0.035 mm

Slit-lamp evaluation revealed that the lens on the right eye had a small V-shaped tear near its center. In addition, the left lens had a small peripheral tear.

III. Assessment/Plan

The patient was diagnosed as having corneal trauma secondary to lens removal that had resulted in two torn lenses. Such damage is sometimes found in patients who remove their lenses directly from the cornea instead of pushing them down onto the sclera first. She admitted to using her fingernails to pinch the lens off the eye. It was not considered necessary to change the contact lens material in this case, but the patient was reeducated in proper lens removal. She was taught to use only the pads of her fingers for removal. Subsequent follow-up visits were uneventful.

IV. Alternative Management Plan/Summary

When a lens tear occurs it is often soon after the patient has received his or her first pair of soft lenses. As a result of the anxiety and cost involved, this problem can eventually lead to discontinuation of lens wear. Thus a comprehensive education program about careful handling of lenses is essential. Certainly ultrathin lenses in a low minus power can be difficult to handle. Therefore, if patient education does not solve the problem, simply changing to a thicker lens material may be successful. If the patient is very motivated to stay in lenses but persists with the problem of tearing lenses, it may be advisable to consider rigid lenses.

Summary

Hydrogel fitting and evaluation are, for the most part, very straightforward. However, it is important to use and carefully evaluate diagnostic lenses in straight-ahead, superior, and inferior gaze. All patients should be properly educated in how to handle the lenses, and the lens care instructions should be reinforced at all follow-up visits. Likewise, corneal integrity (including fluorescein application to assess staining) should be evaluated at every visit.

4

Hydrogel Lens Care and Compliance

Patricia M. Keech

Ensuring the patient's continued success with hydrogel lenses is integrally related to appropriate lens care and a suitable wearing schedule. In fact, the type of lens care system and the recommended wearing time should be a part of the final contact lens prescription. These components of lens fitting are among the many factors evaluated during the contact lens follow-up process (Fig. 4-1 and box on page 49).

For patients to comply with the recommended regimen of lens wear and lens care, the process of patient education needs to be emphasized during fitting. Compliance with all medical treatments is astonishingly poor, but it is easier if the patient understands the risks and ramifications of noncompliance; and even with better than average compliance, over time the nature of the hydrogel lens can cause some complications as the lens changes and ages. It was postulated that the introduction of disposable lenses and planned replacement options in hydrogel fitting strategies would reduce complications and enhance compliance; however, opportunities for contact lens misuse and abuse still appear clinically. Just as one size does not fit all patients, so one care system is not effective for all. During the prescribing process and subsequent periodical evaluations, the practitioner has an opportunity to reinforce the patient's crucial role in caring for lenses, monitoring eye health, and observing the safest

Group Health Cooperative: Contact Lens Associates
Contact Lens Prescription

Patient Name: _____

Lens Material: _____   Date: _____

	Base Curve	Power	Diameter	CT	Tint	Prism	Edge
OD							
OS							

Care System _____   Wearing Time _____
Expiration Date _____

This prescription is valid for one year after the original date, or until the expiration date, if noted. Any lens dispensed, in order to determine compliance with the prescription, must be verified on the patient's eye by a qualified contact lens practitioner in order to assure proper fit and maintenance of eye health.

DM 1340 (5-91)   (Doctor's signature)

FIGURE 4-1 Contact lens prescription form.

wearing schedule. The doctor must also re-evaluate the patient's eye health and make necessary changes in the contact lens fit or care regimen as needed. The following cases delineate clinical situations in which hydrogel lens care or compliance has influenced the patient's ability to wear contact lenses safely and successfully.

• Case One: Noncompliance

I. Subjective Data

A 30-year-old man with a 12-year history of soft contact lens wear presented wearing only his left lens. He reported an eye infection in his right eye 6 weeks earlier for which he had received treatment from a general practitioner. He was told not to wear the right contact lens. He began experiencing headaches on the right side since discontinuing wear of that lens. He was currently taking Tylenol and using a cold disinfection system (Polyquad) nightly along with weekly enzyme cleanings. He usually wore the contact lenses 17 hours per day and wished to resume that schedule.

II. Objective Data

Visual acuity

OD: Unaided   20/80
OS: Ciba   20/20 −3.50 14.0 (1 year old)

Manifest refraction

OD: −1.75 −0.50 X 120   (20/20)
OS: −2.75 −1.00 X 080   (20/20)

Why Is My Contact Lens Prescription Different from My Glasses Prescription?

The prescription for spectacles, or glasses, usually contains the numbers necessary to grind a lens to correct for nearsightedness, farsightedness, astigmatism, or reading problems. These numbers are generally expressed in diopters. Because the lens does not sit directly on the eye, the shape and size of the lens are not as significant as the power of the lens.

With contact lenses, it is a whole different matter. The fitting of the lens has many variables—including the material chosen, the shape, size, and curvature, and the edge design and center thickness. Each of these factors can directly affect the lens performance and how it relates to your eyes. The physiological effect of the contact lens on the eye must be evaluated for a minimum of 2 to 3 months, to determine if contact lens wear is safe for you. *Thus a contact lens prescription cannot be written until the entire fitting process is completed.*

Whenever a contact lens is replaced, the new lens may vary significantly from the old one. As many as 1 in 10 contact lenses is rejected for defects that may not be apparent until they are examined on the eye. That is why we require an inspection of the contact lens on the patient's eye by a qualified practitioner before it is dispensed, both for new fits and for replacements. Therefore a contact lens prescription looks very different from a glasses prescription, and is determined very differently.

To determine if you are a good candidate for contact lens wear, a thorough preliminary examination must be performed. During this examination, the doctor evaluates the physical structures of your eyes, your tear film, your visual needs, and your corrective requirements. If you are a good candidate, the fitting process can begin. Remember: Being fitted with contact lenses is a process that usually takes 2 to 3 months. Annual visits are required after the initial fitting.

Keratometry

OD: 43.75 DS (smooth mires)
OS: 44.00 @ 180; 43.75 @ 090 (smooth mires)

Biomicroscopy

The left contact lens centered with adequate movement but demonstrated advanced protein coating. Both corneas were free of any staining with fluorescein dye. The upper tarsal plates showed a uniform satin appearance with no papillae or follicles. Lids and lashes were clear.

Because the left contact lens was moderately coated, and with a history of eye infection, it was decided to refit with a planned-replacement hydrogel. Optima FW lenses were selected for both eyes with anticipated replacement in 6 months. Lens care and hygiene were reviewed, and it was decided to stay with the Optifree system. The patient failed to return for a scheduled checkup appointment at 2 weeks.

Two months later he presented with a photophobic burning right eye of 3 days' duration.

Visual acuity

OD: Unaided   20/50
 OS: Optima FW   20/20–3

Biomicroscopy

The right eye demonstrated central punctate staining with two 0.5 mm perilimbal infiltrates at 5 o'clock. There was 2+ limbal injection with 2+ flare and cells. The infiltrates did not stain.

Diagnosis: Infiltrative keratitis with iritis OD.

Treatment: Discontinue contact lens wear OD, Tobrex q2h, 5% homatropine tid, 1% prednisolone q4h, follow-up on days 2, 4, and 20.

The patient returned 1 month later for a right lens replacement. He was still wearing only his left lens and refused to wear glasses. He noted that his left eye was not irritated.

Visual acuity

OD: Unaided   20/40 pinhole
 OS: Optima FW   20/20–1

Biomicroscopy

The right eye was clear. The left eye showed a clinical picture similar to that of the right eye 1 month earlier. The inferior limbus demonstrated 2+ limbal injection with several small, discrete, round nonstaining infiltrates from 6 to 9 o'clock. However, the anterior chamber was clear.

III. Assessment/Plan

This type of infiltrative keratoconjunctivitis is generally caused by a hypersensitivity reaction to toxins that accumulate under a tight lens. The time course and eventual involvement of both eyes, as well as the location of the irritation, point to this etiology. Hypersensitivity to the preservatives in care products can also contribute, although then the affected area tends to be more uniform and quickly becomes bilateral.

Since this patient refused to return to spectacles, it was decided to refit the healthy right eye using a preservative-free care system. Because the episode in the left eye was not as clinically advanced as that in the right had been, treatment at this time was limited to contact lens removal and follow-up in 3 days. The right eye was refitted with an 8.60 –2.00 13.8 CSI-T. This lens material was selected for its deposit resistance and oxygen transmission. The fit also allowed more than adequate movement to minimize recurrence of a tight lens. The patient returned for follow-up care 3 days later and 1 week later. The left eye was then refitted with the same CSI-T lens design. He was subsequently evaluated 3 months later, 5 months later, and annually without further incident.

IV. Alternative Management Plan/Summary

This patient was typical in his recurrent red eyes and refusal to return to glasses. When such an individual does not return for routine follow-up care during the fitting process, it can be difficult to avoid or solve complications. Certainly the care system prescribed needs to be simple but also effective. When in doubt, it is advisable to use a preservative-free care system (such as those utilizing hydrogen peroxide) and Miraflow as a daily cleaner to eliminate one source of complications. Frequent-replacement lenses may also reduce complications, but the opportunity to lengthen the "safe" wearing time of such lenses is appealing to patients and this often leads to trouble. In such cases using a deposit-resistant material that allows good oxygen transmission can prevent recurrence and result in a very satisfied and loyal patient.

CLINICAL PEARL

When in doubt, it is advisable to use a preservative-free care system (such as those utilizing hydrogen peroxide) and Miraflow as a daily cleaner to eliminate one source of complications.

• Case Two: Superior Limbal Arcuate Keratitis

I. Subjective Data

A 20-year-old Asian undergraduate student reported for his annual contact lens examination wearing Ciba Visitint hydrogel lenses that were approximately 13 months old. He reported that the right lens had felt dry later in the day for the past few weeks. He was using AOSept disinfection regularly. He was in good health and taking no medications.

II. Objective Data

Visual acuity with contact lenses

OD: 20/20
OS: 20/20
Contact lens specifications

		BCR	Power	OAD
OD:	Ciba Visitint	8.90 mm	−2.50 D	13.8 mm
OS:	Ciba Visitint	8.90 mm	−2.50 D	13.8 mm

Manifest refraction

OD: −2.50 DS   (20/20)
OS: −2.50 DS   (20/20)

Keratometry

OD: 43.50 @ 180; 44.00 @ 090 (smooth mires)
OS: 43.50 @ 180; 44.00 @ 090 (smooth mires)

Biomicroscopy

The contact lenses were centered and moving adequately, but the right lens was heavily coated with protein and the left lens was lightly coated. Further questioning revealed that he had replaced the left lens more recently. After lens removal, inside the limbus of the right eye between 10 and 12 o'clock was an opaque whitish line with associated punctate staining. The left eye was clear, as were the upper tarsal plates.

III. Assessment/Plan

Epithelial splitting is commonly associated with the wearing of coated hydrogel lenses. Mild inflammation may accompany this phenomenon, but it appears to be primarily mechanical irritation (Plate 9). Cessation of contact lens wear is usually necessary for healing, but only for a few days. A different lens or edge design is frequently necessary, although sometimes a fresh lens will be sufficient to prevent recurrence.

This patient was instructed to discontinue lens wear and to return for a refitting in 1 week. He was refitted with an 8.60 mm BCR −3.00 D D2LT. Follow-up over the next 2 years has not shown a recurrence, and the lenses were replaced on a timely basis.

IV. Alternative Management Plan/Summary

Epithelial splitting, or superior limbal arcuate keratitis, in my clinical experience is more common among Asian patients. Anatomical lid considerations support the theory that this is a mechanical phenomenon. When refitting is attempted, an alternate edge design should be employed and usually a smaller steeper lens is selected.

Spoiled lenses also increase the incidence of limbal keratitis, which may be asymptomatic or the patient may describe more "dryness" than usual. Therefore disposable or planned-replacement modalities would also be beneficial in managing this entity. However, the fit of the lens can be crucial and the splitting may recur very quickly if the lens used is inappropriate. Once again, follow-up is necessary to ensure that the hydrogel lenses are fitting appropriately.

Linear punctate staining is sometimes a precursor to actual epithelial splitting. This clinical sign may be missed if the practitioner is not in the habit of staining all soft lens patients at every follow-up examination. It is also necessary to lift the lid to appreciate the condition.

Routine lid eversion and fluorescein staining should be the rule in hydrogel lens follow-up. If these are conscientiously done, the practitioner will be able to prevent many interruptions of lens wear by diagnosing complications at an earlier stage.

CLINICAL PEARL

Routine lid eversion and fluorescein staining should be the rule in hydrogel lens follow-up.

• Case Three: Limbal Epithelial Hypertrophy/Compression

I. Subjective Data

A 27-year-old woman who had worn soft contact lenses for 10 years presented for an initial examination. She was experiencing redness and irritation in her right eye and had noticed decreased vision at distance in both eyes for approximately a week. She was using the Optifree disinfection system with weekly enzyme cleaning but had been unable to wear her right lens on two occasions during the last week due to discomfort. She reported that she was taking no medications and was in good health. The right lens was 7 months old and the left lens about a year old.

II. Objective Data

Visual acuity with contact lenses

		Power	OAD
OD:	Unknown soft lens 20/50	−4.62 D	13.5 mm
OS:	Unknown soft lens 20/40	−4.87 D	13.5 mm

Manifest refraction

OD: −6.50 DS (20/20)
OS: −6.00 −0.50 X 155 (20/20−1)

Keratometry

OD: 45.00 @ 180; 46.00 @ 090 (smooth mires)
OS: 44.75 @ 180; 45.50 @ 090 (smooth mires)

Biomicroscopy

Both contact lenses centered and exhibited advanced protein coating. After lens removal, the right eye showed 2+ limbal injection with hyperemia of the limbal vessels and 1 mm of apparent neovascularization in all quadrants of the cornea. There was also punctate staining overlying the limbal area, with what has been described by Kame[1] as epithelial hypertrophy (that is, elevation and chemosis of the limbal cornea). The central cornea showed subepithelial edema with optic section, but there was no central staining of the right cornea. At 5 o'clock in the peripheral cornea a circular macular scar was noted. The left eye showed some limbal hyperemia and elevation at the 12 o'clock position. The left cornea did not stain and did not appear to be injected. The lids and lashes were clear, as were both upper tarsal plates.

III. Assessment/Plan

Because hydrogel lenses are worn for a relatively long period, the biofilm that is retained on the lens can serve as an attachment for microorganisms. The lens parameters may also be altered, and dehydration can occur more rapidly. Complications may then result from this now "tight" lens. If fluorescein staining is routinely performed, limbal epithelial hypertrophy (or limbal compression) may be appreciated before a red eye occurs. In its early stages an annular thin line of dye pooling just inside the limbus can be noted. Such a finding indicates that the fit may be too tight or the lens needs to be replaced.

This patient was instructed to discontinue lens wear so the inflammation could resolve. She was then refitted with planned-replacement hydrogel lenses using a preservative-free disinfection system (oxidative). Although epithelial hypertrophy is usually associated with extended wear, she was not wearing lenses on an extended-wear basis.

IV. Alternative Management Plan/Summary

In this case patient education needed to emphasize the patient's role in monitoring eye health. An uncomfortable hydrogel lens should not have been worn. At the first sign of persistent redness, tearing, or photophobia, the patient should notify the practitioner's office. At the conclusion of fitting any patient with hydrogel lenses, the doctor needs to inform the patient how long the lenses should last; that is, there should be a definite expiration date on the prescription.

CLINICAL PEARL

At the first sign of persistent redness, tearing, or photophobia, the patient should notify the practitioner's office.

• Case Four: Solution Compliance

I. Subjective Data

A 38-year-old man who had worn soft lenses for 4 years came into the office for an initial evaluation. He had been noticing deposits on his lenses, which were only 4 months old, and also that his eyes were getting red in the afternoon. He normally wore his lenses 16 hours per day. He was storing and rinsing them in saline, using no daily cleaner, and was enzyming weekly.

II. Objective Data

Visual acuity with contact lenses

OD: Unknown soft lens 20/20–1
OS: Unknown soft lens 20/40

Manifest refraction

OD: −3.00 −0.25 X 090 (20/20)
OS: −3.50 DS (20/20)

Keratometry

OD: 46.75 @ 180; 47.25 @ 090 (smooth mires)
OS: 46.75 @ 180; 47.25 @ 090 (smooth mires)

Biomicroscopy

Both hydrogel lenses appeared to be heavily coated. After removal, the corneas demonstrated central, diffuse, and superficial punctate staining with superior limbal injection. The lashes were clear of any debris, but the upper tarsal plates both had a nonuniform cobblestone appearance with papillae less than 0.5 mm in size.

III. Assessment/Plan

Both hydrogel lenses had deposits on them. A mild superficial punctate keratopathy was present from wearing soiled lenses. The patient had not been using any surfactant cleaner or disinfection system. Many patients are confused and believe that enzyme cleaning is, in fact, disinfection.

This man was refitted with quarterly planned-replacement lenses and introduced to a chemical disinfection system with surfactant cleaner and enzyme (Optifree). Follow-up visits 2 weeks and 1 year later showed better compliance and no problems with contact lens wear.

IV. Alternative Management Plan/Summary

Patient education is crucial to successful hydrogel lens care and wearing. The initial training in this case was not adequate, since the patient had acquired bad habits or failed to remember the initial instructions. At every subsequent visit the patient should be asked to review the products that are being used, and how they are being used, to clear up any misconceptions.

CLINICAL PEARL

At every subsequent visit the patient should be asked to review the products that are being used, and how they are being used, to clear up any misconceptions.

• Case Five: Solution Hypersensitivity

I. Subjective Data

A 15-year-old boy presented for an annual eye examination desiring to be fitted with soft contact lenses. He had been previously unsuccessful with rigid gas-permeable (RGP) lenses. He was in good health and taking no medications.

II. Objective Data

Visual acuity (with spectacles)

OD: 20/20
OS: 20/20

Manifest refraction

OD: −4.75 DS (20/20)
OS: −4.75 DS (20/20)

Keratometry

OD: 44.75 @ 180; 45.25 @ 090 (smooth mires)
OS: 44.00 @ 180; 44.75 @ 090 (smooth mires)

Biomicroscopy

The lids and lashes were clear. The corneas were clear and showed no staining with fluorescein. The upper tarsal plates were satin. The tear film break-up time (B.U.T.) was greater than 10 seconds, with adequate tear lake and viscosity. The anterior chambers were deep and clear.

The patient was fitted with Focus planned-replacement lenses for quarterly replacement. The Optifree care system was prescribed. He returned for a 2-week follow-up visit without incident. However, 6 weeks later, at the routine follow-up, he had red eyes.

Visual acuity with contact lenses

OD: 20/25
OS: 20/25

Biomicroscopy

Both eyes showed moderate superficial conjunctival injection. After lens removal, there were symmetrical 360-degree limbal follicles and infiltrates, with trace superficial punctate keratitis. The anterior chambers were clear.

III. Assessment/Plan

This allergic keratoconjunctivitis most probably was a delayed hypersensitivity reaction to the chemical disinfectant. The patient was advised to discontinue contact lens wear and to return in 1 week. At that time, all signs and symptoms were gone. Contact lens wear was reinstituted with a change to preservative-free oxidative system (AOSept). There has been no recurrence during the past 3 years.

IV. Alternative Management Plan/Summary

Whereas infectious processes are generally unilateral, delayed hypersensitivity is most commonly bilateral. Due to improved chemical disinfectants, this type of reaction is not as frequently seen now as it was a decade ago but it does still occur (Plate 10). In some cases a similar clinical picture may result from a toxic reaction, because the concentration of certain preservatives increases in hydrogel lenses over time. More frequent replacement of hydrogel lenses can prevent this scenario.

• Case Six: Giant Papillary Conjunctivitis

I. Subjective Data

A 17-year-old boy who had worn soft contact lenses for 3 years presented for his annual examination wearing the left lens only; the right one had been lost 3 days earlier. His lenses were approximately a year old. He reported that for the last few weeks they had been moving around more than usual and he was experiencing some itching in both eyes. He was in good health and taking no medications. The Optifree disinfection system was what he normally used to clean his lenses.

II. Objective Data

Visual acuity

OD: Unaided 20/400
OS: Vantage 20/40 (with 8.9 mm BCR, −4.50 D, 14.0 mm OAD)

Manifest refraction

OD: −5.25 −0.50 X 030 (20/20)
OS: −4.50 DS (20/20)

Biomicroscopy

The left lens was extremely coated and had a greasy appearance. It moved excessively (2+ mm) with the blink. After removal, the cornea exhibited central punctate staining and the upper tarsal plates had moderate papillae OU without active mucus secretion. The right eye did not show any fluorescein staining. There was minimal injection of the bulbar conjunctiva OU.

III. Assessment/Plan

Giant papillary conjunctivitis (GPC), a hypersensitivity response to the denatured protein on a soiled contact lens, with attendant increased mucus production, was apparent in this case. Because the papillae were moderate in size with no active visible mucus accumulation, it was decided to refit and replace without stopping contact lens wear. The lenses selected were Seequence II for daily wear with monthly replacement. The care system was switched to Ultracare (an oxidative system) to avoid preservatives.

IV. Alternative Management Plan/Summary

In cases of GPC it is frequently necessary to interrupt contact lens wear to break the cycle of hypersensitivity responses. Generally, if the papillae have mucus attached to them or if the size and number of papillae are excessive (grade 3 or 4), a minimum 2-week cessation of lens wear is indicated.

Extended-wear schedules are inadvisable for patients with a history of GPC. Planned-replacement lenses are one method of managing this entity. Another, very workable, option is to select a more deposit-resistant hydrogel material (such as Crofilcon A). In any case, the patient must be completely retrained in lens care and hygiene, emphasizing the importance of all the elements—surfactant cleaning, disinfection, and enzyme cleaning. Follow-up appointments at regular intervals also aid in preventing recurrence at an earlier stage, and in some cases switching to RGP lenses is a solution.

• Case Seven: Make-up with Extended Wear

I. Subjective Data

A 52-year-old woman presented with extended-wear disposable soft contact lenses that she had been changing on a weekly basis. She reported using one eye for distance and the other for near but found that her lenses were becoming foggy before the end of the week. She had been using disposable lenses for approximately a year, was taking no medications or eye drops, and appeared to be in good health.

II. Objective Data

Visual acuity with contact lenses

OD: Newvue 20/50 (near)
OS: Newvue 20/25 (distance)

Overrefraction

OD: +0.50 D 20/40 (near)
OS: Plano 20/25 (distance)

Manifest refraction

OD: +1.00 DS 20/20
OS: +1.00 DS 20/20

Biomicroscopy

Both lenses centered and moved adequately. The left lens had a small peripheral crack over the limbal area, of which the patient was unaware. Both lenses had accumulations of small black specks in addition to moderate protein coating. The patient had copious amounts of mascara on her lashes. After lens removal, the corneas did not stain with fluorescein and there was no significant corneal edema. The upper tarsal plates had a uniform cobblestone appearance. The tear viscosity was grade 3, with excessive debris in the tear film.

III. Assessment/Plan

In this case the generous use of cosmetics appeared to be affecting the performance of the patient's contact lenses. High-viscosity tears can also result from using oily cosmetic-removal products. The patient was instructed to remove all mascara (preferably water soluble) every night using a nonoily remover. Diluted baby shampoo was suggested since it works well, as do lid scrub products (for example, Lids and Lashes). She was told never to apply eyeliner posterior to the lash line.

The patient chose to return to daily wear with a planned-replacement lens. With daily cleaning it is usually preferable to insert the contact lenses before applying makeup and to remove them before cosmetic removal. This will minimize lens spoilage.

IV. Alternative Management Plan/Summary

The use of cosmetics with extended-wear lenses is a delicate situation. For optimal condition of the lids and lashes, complete removal of makeup each night is required; but the products used must be oil-free to avoid disrupting meibomian gland function. Contamination can also occur from infected products. Mascara should be replaced frequently, approximately every 3 months. Lens cases should be rinsed to eliminate any pathogens. With daily wear it is advisable to rinse the case when a lens is inserted in the morning, allow the case to air dry during the day, and use fresh disinfection solution each night.

> **CLINICAL PEARL**
>
> *With daily wear it is advisable to rinse the case when a lens is inserted in the morning, allow the case to air dry during the day, and use fresh disinfection solution each night.*

• Case Eight: Overwear

I. Subjective Data

A 24-year-old woman presented on an emergency basis with the complaint of a teary photophobic left eye for the past 24 hours. She normally wore disposable contact lenses for 2 weeks at a time, replacing them each time she took them out. She reported having had a similar incident 6 months earlier and also that she had dry eye problems. She did not bring her lenses to this visit and had not worn them since the previous day. She was in good health otherwise and was currently taking no medications.

II. Objective Data

Visual acuity with habitual spectacle correction

OD: 20/20   (−8.75 −0.50 X 003)
OS: 20/20−3   (−9.87 −0.25 X 066)

Biomicroscopy

The left eye demonstrated 2+ limbal injection, 1+ flare and cells, and no hypopyon in the anterior chamber. The pupils were reactive to light directly and consensually. There was a circular well-defined corneal infiltrate near the limbus at 7 o'clock OS less than 1 mm in size. The right eye was clear. In the left eye two circular small macular scars were noted near the limbus at 1:30. The infiltrate in the left eye did not stain with fluorescein.

Noncontact tonometry (mm Hg at 12:15 PM)

OD: 14
OS: 12

III. Assessment/Plan

Marginal infiltrative keratitis in the left eye and a mild iritis associated with overwear of hydrogel contact lenses were present. The scarring of the left cornea and the history suggested that this problem was recurrent. The keratitis was treated with Tobrex ophthalmic solution q2h OS. The left eye was dilated with 5% homatropine. Follow-up visits at 1 and 4 days showed acceptable resolution.

Due to the repetitive nature of this inflammation, the advisability of extended wear for such a patient might be called into question. Especially with a history of "dry eye" symptomatology and a highly myopic prescription, the appropriateness of an extended-wear schedule should be reevaluated. After complete resolution of the inflammation, the fit of the contacts would need to be evaluated with particular attention to satisfying the physiological requirements for this patient. Daily-wear soft lenses or RGP lenses would be two options to consider. In high prescriptions, wearing an extended-wear lens on a daily basis might be required to allow adequate oxygen transmission for this patient's corneas. Corneal hypoxia has been shown to create an environment that favors infection and inflammation.

CLINICAL PEARL

Especially with a history of "dry eye" symptomatology and a highly myopic prescription, the appropriateness of an extended-wear schedule should be reevaluated.

IV. Alternative Management Plan/Summary

Certain lens designs have superior efficacy in such cases of high myopia with exceptional oxygen requirements. If a soft lens is required, the CSI-T design and HO4 seem to provide the best results in my experience.

Summary

One of the most important elements in prescribing hydrogel lenses is to educate the patient regarding appropriate lens care, wearing schedules, and the necessity of regular consultations. Wearing contact lenses is a dynamic sequence of events. The lenses change with time, as do the eyes. Follow-up appointments are a great opportunity to review solutions and their use, the symptoms to be alert for, and how the patient is utilizing the lenses.

Although the U.S. Food and Drug Administration has approved some hydrogel lenses for 7-day continuous wear, the physiological requirements of patients vary and recommended wearing schedules need to be developed for each person. Informing the patient of the risks of extended wear is also part of the educational process.

The earliest symptoms of serious eye infections associated with hydrogel lens wear have been shown to be persistent photophobia and tearing. All hydrogel lens wearers need to be informed that if they experience any persistent discomfort the contact lens must be removed and the eye doctor contacted immediately.

Straightforward hygiene will minimize contamination of soft contact lenses. Clean hands and clean cases can prevent many complications. Again, these concepts should be reviewed with the patient at regular follow-up visits.

The array of hydrogel lens care products has expanded and improved over the last several years, as have the types of lenses available. However, patient compliance continues to be a challenge as the options become more confusing. The contact lens practitioner's role is crucial in educating the patient and prescribing not just lenses but appropriate care systems and wearing schedules.

Bibliography

1. Kame RT: Limbal epithelial hypertrophy. *Int Contact Lens Clin* 14(11):453, 1987.

5

Disposable Lenses

Ian M. Lane

Disposable contact lenses have provided us with an effective tool in compliance management. Compliance has always been one of the primary challenges in our field. There is little doubt that complications secondary to contact lens wear would be far less of an issue if patients followed lens wear and care instructions better. Indeed, a majority of the complications we see clinically are related to poor compliance.

Non-compliance can be divided into three categories:

1. Wear schedule
2. Appointments (not kept by the patient or not scheduled by the doctor)
3. Solutions

Wear Schedule

Wear schedule compliance is a function of patient education and consistent and repeated reinforcement by the practitioner and staff. We have all heard the patient who says "... but doctor the lenses are so comfortable I just assumed everything was all right." It is part of our job to educate these individuals that contact lenses, and particularly extended-wear lenses, are not cosmetic but rather are medical devices that provide clear vision and are generally safe when used as directed. We must emphasize that comfort and vision are not reliable predictors of continued success. There is certainly a cosmetic phase to lens wear, but long-term cosmetic success cannot be accomplished in the absence of long-term ocular health.

Appointment Compliance

Extended wear means extended care. The partnership between patient and provider is a key factor in long-term success. We begin with the premise that patients want to comply. However, patients in the 1990s want the most health without sacrificing convenience. Since compliance is a function of education, we can reinforce the combining of these not necessarily compatible entities by sending a clear message of how much importance we place on follow-up care by scheduling the next appointment at the conclusion of each visit. This appointment must be administered by the office staff; reminder phone calls or cards should be a part of the daily office routine.

Solutions

The pharmaceutical industry has developed products in an attempt to simplify lens care while maintaining safety and efficacy for our patients. Despite their efforts, however, the hygiene regimen has remained too complicated and time consuming. What is needed is a fresh approach to contact lens care. If the environment were such that lenses could be discarded consistently, the complication rate might go down; and experience has shown this to be the case. Nevertheless, even then, disposability would not replace regular follow-up care by the doctor. Although it could reduce many of the complications that affect case management associated with ordinary reuseable contact lenses, there would still be the need for appropriate lens selection and fitting.

Following are selected cases that demonstrate the clinical elements in which the prescription of disposable contact lenses influenced the case prognosis positively.

• Case One: Seborrheic Dermatitis/Blepharitis

I. Subjective Data

A 28-year-old certified public accountant presented to our office with a long history of seborrheic dermatitis and blepharitis. He had been attempting to wear contact lenses (rigid gas-permeable, hydrogel, daily- and extended-wear) for several years but had not had much success.

II. Objective Data

Visual acuity uncorrected

OD: 20/400
OS: 20/400

Manifest refraction

OD: −4.25 DS (20/20)
OS: −4.25 DS (20/20)

Keratometry

OD: 43.87 @ 180; 44.12 @ 090 (mires clear and regular)
OS: 43.75 @ 180; 44.12 @ 090 (mires clear and regular)

Biomicroscopy

Biomicroscopy confirmed the presence of a marginal blepharitis OU, with typical lid margin flush and flakes between the cilia. The conjunctiva also revealed the typical dull red flush of blepharitis. The tears had floating debris from flakes that had dropped into the lacrimal fluid. A slight photophobia was detected during slit-lamp examination.

Because this patient represented his company publicly, he was particularly concerned about his appearance with spectacles. He was also concerned over the appearance of his lids and eyes in general. He frequently had to remove his spectacles to rub his eyes when they became itchy, and the questions from colleagues and clients as to whether he was feeling ill embarrassed him. He had been treated for the dermatitis and blepharitis; but since these appeared to be associated with his stress level and were recurring, his compliance with the medications and contact lens cleaning had begun to deteriorate over time.

III. Assessment/Plan

In view of the recurrent nature of this condition, it was decided that the patient needed to be thoroughly indoctrinated in its characteristics. Ongoing and continuous care would have to become a part of his life. The sequelae of noncompliance were emphasized. During the instruction he disclosed that this was the first time anyone had explained to him the reasons for ongoing treatment; he now understood his condition and would be a more active participant in its management.

Lid scrubs bid were recommended for 2 weeks. If the lid condition improved, a lens-wear regimen would be introduced with frequent follow-up examinations.

When the patient presented 2 weeks later, his lids were markedly improved and the flakes between the cilia were virtually absent. The debris in the lacrimal fluid was almost nonexistent. He was extremely motivated because of the short-term improvement. Based on these encouraging results we decided to proceed with a contact lens fitting. Once again, ongoing management was emphasized.

The goal of the fitting was to use a disposable lens in a daily-wear regimen with a weekly or more frequent discard cycle based (at least initially) on the following rationale:

1. If the lenses were discarded regularly, this would reduce the amount of time he had to spend on care of the materials.
2. Daily wear was essential as long as debris was likely to be present in the lacrimal fluid. Hypersensitivity reactions due to debris entrapment could thereby be avoided.
3. Lid scrubs would be continued bid and then tapered to ad as long as the condition of the lids remained quiet. The frequency of lid scrubs could be increased by any onset of hyperemia.
4. A hydrogel lens with limbus-to-limbus coverage would protect the cornea from blepharitic epidermal cells that might come into contact with the cornea. The symptoms of burning, itching, and photophobia could thereby be reduced.
5. In the long term, if he was free of symptoms and clinical signs, a return to flexible extended-wear lenses could be considered (although this was unlikely). (In fact, the patient built up his wearing time to a comfortable 16 hours per day.)

Because the recurrences of blepharitis and dermatological conditions are unpredictable, I recommended a true daily-wear disposable lens for this patient. Since then, unscheduled office visits have been eliminated. He also enjoys not having to worry about any cleaning or disinfecting whatsoever, and his wearing time has increased to cover all his waking hours. The seborrheic dermatitis is treated with 0.5% hydrocortisone prn.

Thus, whereas he initially discontinued lens wear on a weekly basis because of the time and effort involved, he now merely discards his lenses daily. He has periodical episodes of active blepharitis apparently secondary to, or in association with, an outbreak of seborrhea. He has recently sought care from a dermatologist, who prescribed a 0.5% hydrocortisone liquid to reduce the inflammation on the cheeks and Blephamide for the lids as necessary. I currently reexamine him at 6-month intervals. It is apparent that compliance is the key to ongoing success, and patient communication/education is the key to compliance.

IV. Alternative Management Plan/Summary

Other options for this patient would be as follows:
1. Cease contact lens wear altogether and return to spectacles.
2. Daily wear/monthly replacement with medical treatment. This was not considered the highest level of care because of the patient's previous record of solution and medication compliance.

3. Refractive surgery. This also was not actively considered because the patient was fearful of having to undergo any kind of operative intervention.

• Case Two: Latent Hyperopia

I. Subjective Data

A 33-year-old software engineer presented to the office with a history of chronic headaches. He had been using analgesics frequently for several years. Apparently an etiology could not be found. Previous doctors had virtually given up and as much as told him he would have to learn to live with his symptoms. He was wearing spectacles for near, but they only periodically helped. His general health was good, and his family history unremarkable.

II. Objective Data

Habitual spectacle prescription

OD: +0.75 DS
OS: +0.75 DS

Uncorrected distance visual acuity

OD: 20/25
OS: 20/25
OU: 20/25

Retinoscopy

+3.00 DS OU

The results varied from +0.50 to +3.50 D, and the retinosopic reflex changed during the procedure.

Cycloplegic refraction

OD: +3.75 DS (20/20)
OS: +4.00 DS (20/20)

Keratometry

OD: 43.50 @ 017; 44.62 @ 107 (mires clear and regular)
OS: 44.00 @ 172; 44.75 @ 082 (mires clear and regular)

Manifest refraction

OD: +1.25 DS (20/20, variable)
OS: +1.75 DS (20/20, variable)

Biomicroscopy

The anterior external examination was unremarkable OU, the pupils appearing to be smaller than expected for a patient of this age.

III. Assessment/Plan

This patient was diagnosed as having latent hyperopia and asthenopia. I recommended contact lenses for full-time wear, and possibly extended wear if physiologically feasible, to reduce his ability to remove the prescription for even short periods. The maximum tolerated plus was introduced immediately and was then increased as indicated by manifest refraction and stability of the retinoscopic reflex.

CLINICAL PEARL

Disposable extended-wear lenses were recommended to reduce the costs to the patient as the powers were changed to accommodate his rehabilitation from latent to manifest hyperopia.

Disposable extended-wear lenses were recommended to reduce the costs to the patient as the powers were changed to accommodate his rehabilitation from latent to manifest hyperopia. In addition, experience has taught us that latent hyperopes are traditionally not very happy at first because of their variable visual acuity and our inability to immediately "cure" the problem. We felt it more appropriate to reduce the amount of "extraneous things" this patient would have to do in caring for his lenses. After all, his primary goal was cessation of the discomfort and visual acuity and secondarily, not to wear glasses.

Initial contact lens prescription

			BCR	OAD	Power
(9/26/90)	OD:	Acuvue	9.1 mm	14.4 mm	+1.50 D
	OS:	Acuvue	9.1 mm	14.4 mm	+2.00 D

Subsequent contact lens prescriptions

(10/31/90)	OD:	Acuvue	9.1 mm	14.4 mm	+2.50 D
	OS:	Acuvue	9.1 mm	14.4 mm	+2.75 D
(8/28/91)	OD:	Acuvue	9.1 mm	14.4 mm	+3.00 D
	OS:	Acuvue	9.1 mm	14.4 mm	+2.75 D
(3/4/92)	OD:	Acuvue	9.1 mm	14.4 mm	+3.00 D (no change)
	OS:	Acuvue	9.1 mm	14.4 mm	+3.25 D

(7/7/93) A cycloplegic refraction was performed because he was again presenting mild symptoms of asthenopia. At this visit it was decided to prescribe the refraction in the lenses minus 0.75 D for tonus in the accommodative system. The patient would also be examined on a daily basis for several days as the cycloplegic effects diminished.

OD:	Acuvue	9.1 mm	14.4 mm	+3.25 D
OS:	Acuvue	9.1 mm	14.4 mm	+3.25 D (no change)

Repeated refractions over the next few days were stable, and the visual acuity remained 20/20 for both distance and near.

IV. Alternative Management Plan/Summary

Other options included the following:
1. Bifocal spectacles initially. This was not implemented because
   a. The patient did not like the idea of bifocals/multifocals since he had not performed well with glasses in the past.
   b. He felt that bifocals would "age him."
   c. The potential of visual changes made Acuvue contact lenses more cost effective.
2. Spectacles in combination with visual training. Visual training was discussed, but the patient believed he did not want to make the time commitment.
3. Contact lenses in combination with reading spectacles (with or without visual training). He did not like the idea of wearing spectacles.

The patient was first fitted in 1990 and has continued to wear lenses successfully since that time. The discard cycle was set to be every 2 weeks initially, with weekly removal for cleaning and disinfection, but was shorted to weekly because there was evidence of a few microcysts in each eye at the last annual eye examination. Although arguable that this might be acceptable clinically, I elected to reduce the usage time to 1 week only. As of his most recent progress evaluation, all microcysts had resolved in each eye. His refraction has remained stable since then and all symptoms have resolved. He no longer uses analgesics to get him through the day.

• Case Three: Occupational Hygiene

I. Subjective Data

A 57-year-old dentist who had previously worn reusable extended-wear lenses was referred to our office by a colleague for his annual eye health and vision examination. He was motivated to consider disposable contact lenses for hygiene purposes because in his profession there could be flying oral debris.

II. Objective Data

Manifest refraction

OD: −2.50 DS   (20/20) add +2.00 D (20/20)
OS: −2.75 DS   (20/20) add +2.00 D (20/20)

Keratometry

OD: 43.12 @ 180; 42.62 @ 090 (mires clear and regular)
OS: 43.12 @ 180; 42.62 @ 090 (mires clear and regular)

Biomicroscopy

Anterior external examination was unremarkable OU.

III. Assessment/Plan

This patient was a simple myope with presbyopia. Because of the nature of his profession, he worked at closer than normal distances, and he desired to continue wearing contact lenses but was happy to have a spectacle overcorrection as well. I recommended true daily-wear disposable lenses to further reduce his apprehension about possible contamination from oral debris and to decrease the number of extended-wear office visits he would have to make. A spectacle overprescription, designed for comfort at his usual working distance and as a further shield against flying debris, and a pair of reading glasses with an add appropriate for normal reading conditions were prescribed.

Contact lens prescription

OD: Acuvue   −2.50 D   (20/20)
OS: Acuvue   −2.50 D   (20/20)

Spectacle prescription

Occupational: with a higher add (+3.25 DS) OU
Regular near vision: with an add (+2.00 DS) OU

IV. Alternative Management Plan/Summary

Other options included
1. Glasses (bifocals/progressives) initially. This was not implemented because he was already a satisfied contact lens wearer. His goal was to further reduce the risk of contamination and infection as a result of his profession.
2. Frequent-replacement lenses. Neither he nor I felt that these would be as effective in terms of reaching his goal of having the "safest" mode of protection in his capacity as a dentist.

He was fitted with Acuvue true daily-wear disposable lenses in January of 1992 and has continued to wear them successfully since then. The daily discard cycle proved to lower his apprehension over the possibility of contamination during treatment of patients. In addition, he has been extremely satisfied with the convenience of a daily discard cycle.

• Case Four: Alternating Esotropia and Presbyopia

I. Subjective Data

A 45-year-old administrator who was recently relocated to the West Coast expressed concern over her right eye, which tended to turn in. She believed it was more pronounced when she wore spectacles because of the magnification by the convex lenses. She had experienced the problem since childhood, but because her left eye had good distance vision she was not motivated to wear glasses. She had always believed that her vision was fine despite the fact that, after accepting the job, she had begun to notice her vision becoming blurry. She also complained of headaches, usually around midday. In addition, her right eye appeared to turn in more now than she remembered.

She had consistently not worn her glasses because she did not like to be seen in them. She also indicated that when she wore them she noticed no improvement in binocular vision. Her general health was good, and she was not experiencing any allergies or taking any medications.

II. Objective Data

Uncorrected visual acuity

OD: 20/100
OS: 20/20

The refraction showed hyperopia, presbyopia, and alternating esotropia (OS dominant).

Manifest refraction

OD: +1.75 DS (20/20) add +1.50 (20/25)
OS: +0.50 DS (20/20) add +1.50 (20/25)

Keratometry

OD: 42.25 @ 180; 42.37 @ 090 (mires clear and regular)
OS: 42.87 @ 180; 43.00 @ 090 (mires clear and regular)

Biomicroscopy

The anterior external examination was unremarkable in each eye.

III. Assessment/Plan

This patient was a hyperopic accommodative esotrope with presbyopia. I recommended disposable contact lenses in a monovision prescription. Because her right eye was nondominant, it was prescribed for near. She was not binocular but was correctable to 20/25, so I thought it important to optimize the function of this eye. The goal was to meet her needs of not wearing glasses and at the same time improve her visual acuity for both distance and near.

Contact lens prescription

		Power	Visual acuity
OD:	Acuvue	+3.75	(20/20, near)
OS:	Acuvue	+0.50	(20/20, distance)

Her visual adaptation was almost immediate. She reported that after the first day she was completely asymptomatic, with both physical comfort and ease of handling the lenses. Her wearing time was gradually increased to 6 consecutive nights, with weekly monitoring for the first 2 months. Follow-up visits consisted of inspecting her corneal physiology (particularly OD) for signs of hypoxic stress. One straie was detected centrally in this eye, as would be expected because of the thicker lens profile and corresponding reduction in the Dk/L. It was temporary and has not been observed since.

Of particular interest in this case was the fact that both distance and near visual acuities in her right eye were improved to 20/20 from 20/25 at the 6-month progress evaluation. She commented that the lenses felt so much a part of her she could not remember what her vision had been like all those years when she was refusing to wear glasses. She currently was being checked every 6 months and continued to wear the disposable extended-wear lenses with a 1-week wear time and discard every 2 weeks. Her prescription had changed and now was

		BCR	OAD	Power
OD:	Acuvue	9.1 mm	14.4 mm	+4.00 D (near, 20/20)
OS:	Acuvue	9.1 mm	14.4 mm	+1.25 D (distance, 20/20)

IV. Alternative Management Plan/Summary

Four options were available for this patient:
1. Binocular contact lenses for distance acuity with spectacle correction for reading. This was not recommended because of her consistent avoidance of glasses since early childhood.
2. Glasses (bifocal/progressive) initially. This also was not implemented because she had a history of avoiding spectacle wear and appeared to be even more averse to bifocals or multifocals upon presentation of this option to her.
3. Daily-wear frequent-replacement monovision lenses. Upon assessing her temperament, it was my opinion (and she agreed) that these would not be an effective alternative since she was a single working mother with two jobs. The extra time necessary to care for daily-wear lenses might have resulted in her discontinuing lens wear.
4. Extended-wear or daily-wear bifocal/multifocal lenses. It was my opinion that this would not be in her best interest since she was not binocular and there would thus be no summation effect. Furthermore, of the "simultaneous-vision," "alternating-vision," or "combination" presbyopic hydrogel lens designs available today, none provides clinically satisfactory monocular vision in both mesopic and scotoptic conditions.

This case allowed the clinician to take advantage of a less than optimal binocular status and transform it into an asset for the patient. What was essentially a nonfunctioning tropic eye was changed into a functional part of her day-to-day life.

CLINICAL PEARL

In this case we changed what was essentially a nonfunctioning tropic eye into a functional part of the patient's day-to-day life.

• Case Five: Accommodative Esotropia

I. Subjective Data

A 14-year-old girl who had been wearing a spectacle correction from the age of 2 would not wear her glasses in school because they made her appear "bug-eyed." She was originally fitted at age 5 with CSI daily-wear contact lenses but, because of the nature of the CSI material and her immaturity, had experienced many breakages. She was now attending junior high and was, understandably, more concerned than ever about her appearance. Her eye troped as soon as she removed a lens. She was concerned about losing or tearing a lens while at school, and she was particularly shy about sleeping over at her friends' houses because the other girls would ask her about her eyes when she removed her lenses. She and her parents were seeking advice on how to solve this dilemma.

II. Objective Data

Prior contact lens prescription

		BCR	OAD	Power
OD:	CSI	8.6 mm	14.5 mm	+4.75 D
OS:	CSI	8.6 mm	14.5 mm	+5.00 D

Uncorrected visual acuity

OD: 20/100
OS: 20/100

Manifest refraction

The refraction showed a fairly elevated hyperopia with alternating accommodative esotropia.

OD: +5.00 DS (20/20, distance and near)
OS: +4.75 DS (20/20, distance and near)

Keratometry

OD: 43.75 @ 090; 43.50 @ 180 (mires clear and regular)
OS: 43.75 @ 165; 44.37 @ 075 (mires clear and regular)

Biomicroscopy

Anterior external examination of her eyes was unremarkable.

III. Assessment/Plan

This patient was a hyperope with accommodative esotropia. Disposable extended-wear lenses were recommended, provided the high-plus profile did not cause a clinically unacceptable physiological response.

Contact lens prescription

		BCR	OAD	Power
OD:	Acuvue	9.1 mm	14.4 mm	+5.00 D (20/20)
OS:	Acuvue	9.1 mm	14.4 mm	+5.00 D (20/20)

She adapted well to daily wear with a lower–water content lens, immediately initiating overnight wear, and returned the next day for a follow-up appointment. This time was used to check for any residual corneal swelling after she had been awake and in the open-eye situation for several hours. The examination revealed no striae, with good centration and post-blink movement OU. She was rescheduled for another examination on the seventh day, with similar biomicroscopic results. Both she and her parents were pleased that we could meet her needs. It was emphasized that extended-wear lenses are a medical device with a higher risk of complications than is associated with daily-wear. The parents and patient were educated in the "what ifs" of extended-wear and, in particular, the effects of high-plus contact lenses on oxygen transmissibility. We have seen her every 3 months since the original fitting, in 1990.

IV. Alternative Management Plan/Summary

Four options were available for this patient:
1. Ordinary reusable extended-wear lenses. This was rejected because I wanted to reduce the number of steps she would have to go through to maintain her lenses. It has been my experience that the less we require of patients, especially teenagers, the more likely they are to comply with the prescribed regimen.
2. Extended-wear frequent-replacement lenses. This option was rejected for the same reasons.
3. Daily-wear frequent-replacement lenses. This option was rejected because it was one of the problems she had verbalized during the case history (i.e., having to remove her lenses in the presence of friends).
4. Ordinary reusable daily-wear lenses. This was rejected for the same reason.

As of her last visit to the office (12/93) the patient was still asymptomatic. Biomicroscopy revealed clear healthy corneas, with no striae or microcystic response. Her maximum wear time was 6 nights, with a 7-day discard cycle.

• Case Six: Unilateral Myopia with Presbyopia

I. Subjective Data

A 39-year-old woman working as a freelance writer for a boating magazine, who sailed frequently, came to the office with two problems involving long-term RGP lens wear. (1) She wore only one lens, and people commented that the eye with the lens always appeared to be droopy and small. She had been informed by her previous doctor that if she wore a contact lens she would have to accept the "smaller" eye. (2) She was soon to leave on an extended sailing trip (circumnavigating the globe) and was concerned that she might fall asleep with her lens in place. In addition, she had heard that contact lenses could be washed or blown out of the eye in heavy seas, and she wanted to avoid handling the lens as much as possible. The vision with her RGP lens was clear, and her average wearing time was over 10 hours a day.

II. Objective Data

Biomicroscopy

RGP lens fitting appeared to be on alignment, with some residual cylinder manifest. There was mild arcuate staining of the bulbar conjunctiva from 11 to 1 o'clock. This corresponded to the location that the lens would bind at the limit of upward translation during the opening phase of the blink. This was judged to be of no clinical significance. Lid edema was present in her right superior eyelid and was particularly obvious in view of the fact that this was a unilateral fitting. The narrower palpebral fissure was definitely visible, even to the casual observer. The corneas were unremarkable, although the right eye had a classical foreign body track. The tears appeared to be clear and plentiful, with a large lacrimal lake inferiorly.

Manifest refraction

OD: −1.75   −0.25 × 010   (20/20)
OS: Plano   −0.25 × 150   (20/20)

Keratometry

OD: 40.75 @ 009; 41.87 @ 099 (Delta K = −1.12 DC × 009)
OS: 40.25 @ 171; 41.75 @ 081 (Delta K = −1.50 DC × 171)

III. Assessment/Plan

Since she was going to be sailing for a prolonged period, disposable soft contact lenses were proposed as the most suitable modality for her. The benefits of a hydrogel lens would include the following:

1. Reduced lid edema, typical of most RGP fits, which would tend to increase the lid aperture over time. This would also enhance the symmetry of her facial features.
2. A sufficient number of sterile backup lenses. This would address the concern she had over possibly losing a lens at sea.

3. Extended wearing time. This would ensure that if she had to remain awake for a long time (due to foul weather) or had to sleep for a short time she would not have to deal with insertion and removal.
4. Minimal hand contact. This would reduce the chances of contamination, since sailboating does not always provide the best environment for cleanliness.

CLINICAL PEARL
By utilizing a disposable hydrogel lens we can ensure that there will always be a sufficient number of sterile backup lenses available, thereby addressing the concern about lost lenses.

Contact lens prescription

OD: No lens   (20/20)
OS: Acuvue   (8.8 mm BCR, 14.0 mm OAD, −2.25 D) (20/20)

A daily-wear schedule was initiated for 1 week; overnight wear was then initiated, with a progress-check visit at 24 hours, followed by other progress checks at 1, 2, 4, 8, and 10 weeks, and finally one at 3 months until she set sail. We agreed that she would call every 3 months for a phone progress report once she was under way. Throughout this time biomicroscopy was negative. Her final wearing schedule was to be 6 nights, with a weekly discard as long as she remained asymptomatic.

After 5 years she is still wearing her lenses on an extended-wear basis (6 nights) and living in the Caribbean. She comes annually for an eye examination and contact lens evaluation, and we continue to carry on phone progress checks every 6 months unless symptoms are present.

Current spectacle prescription

OD: −2.50   −0.25 × 180
OS: Plano   −0.50 × 175

Overreading spectacle prescription

OD: Add +1.00
OS: Add +1.00 −0.50 × 175

IV. Alternative Management Plan/Summary

Four options were available for this patient:
1. Refit both eyes with rigid gas-permeable (RGP) lenses to obtain symmetry of the lids. This was not pursued, because of her residual astigmatism and her life-style.

2. Refer her to an ophthalmic surgeon for refractive surgery. She was not particularly excited about this option.
3. Prescribe spectacles. Because of her long history of contact lens wear and her upcoming nautical life-style, this was not considered a serious option as a means of correcting her vision. However, she was given a spectacle prescription to have for back-up purposes.
4. Use monovision lenses without correction, since she was a unilateral myope. This was considered, but she had a very dominant right eye and felt most uncomfortable using her left eye for distance viewing.

The program selected was quite successful in meeting all the goals set for this patient. The edema in her right upper lid gradually resolved over time. The palpebral apertures are not identical, but the difference is not noticeable to the casual observer.

• Case Seven: Pinguecula

I. Subjective Data

This 29-year-old woman had been wearing daily-wear Cibasoft lenses (BCR 9.0 mm, OAD 14.5 mm) for about a year. Six months earlier she reported blurriness in one eye to her attending doctor. Upon reexamination, another pair of daily-wear contact lenses was prescribed along with spectacles with a prism correction. This did not solve her unilateral blurry vision problem. She then consulted another doctor, who performed three "trial fits." The problem was still not resolved, and she was referred to an ophthalmologist who, in turn, referred her to our office (in July 1990).

II. Objective Data

The overrefraction disclosed that her visual acuity in the left eye could be improved from 20/60 to 20/20 although the vision was variable. Slit-lamp examination revealed a pinguecula with an unusually raised apex displaced toward the limbus OS. The large-diameter lens (14.5 mm) was being raised by the leading edge of the pinguecula and had been torqued due to the interaction between lid, lens, and uneven conjunctival surface created by the pinguecula. It was speculated that this might be the cause of her variable vision and subjective discomfort. To rule this out, the retinoscopic reflex over the lens in both eyes was observed. The postblink reflex in the left eye showed an oblique (variable) axis with poor optics whereas the right eye had a uniform crisp over-retinoscopic reflex. In addition, a hand-held illuminated Keeler keratoscope was used to observe the quality of the mires over both contact lenses. An oblique axis and variable distorted mires were evident in the left eye. Finally, to rule out an irregular astigmatism OS, a manifest refraction and keratometry were performed.

Manifest refraction

OD: −1.75 −0.25 × 130 (20/20)
OS: −3.75 DS (20/20)

Keratometry

OD: 44.00 @ 180; 45.37 @ 090 (smooth mires)
OS: 44.25 @ 170; 45.25 @ 080 (smooth mires)

Biomicroscopy

The anterior external examination was unremarkable OD. Her left eye manifested an arcuate fluorescein stain corresponding to the position of the lens edge. The stain had a width of 2 mm as measured with the Haag-Streit slit lamp. Mild staining was also present at the apex of the pinguecula.

III. Assessment/Plan

Her variable visual acuity was caused by asymmetrical postblink lens movement secondary to the pinguecula OS. A smaller-diameter lens with a very thin soft edge that would be less affected by her atypical conjunctival topography was fitted on the left eye. Because of the fitting characteristics of Acuvue lenses (which tend to decenter temporally in cases I have observed with pingueculae in the past), these were selected.

Contact lens prescription

		BCR	OAD	Power
OD:	Acuvue	8.8 mm	14.0 mm	−2.25 D (20/20)
OS:	Acuvue	8.8 mm	14.0 mm	−4.00 D (20/20)

The lenses performed exactly as expected and were decentered slightly temporally without sacrificing limbus-to-limbus coverage. With the very thin soft edge there was minimal contact with the pinguecula in the left eye. The patient reported an immediate improvement in comfort. A daily-wear schedule was prescribed, starting at 5 hours on day 1 and adding 2 hours on each successive day. At the 1-week follow-up visit she reported that she was seeing clearly out of each eye. Her eyes felt comfortable and were white. Slit-lamp examination confirmed her subjective report. There were no signs of irritation and her visual acuity remained 20/20 OD, OS, and OU. Very mild fluorescein staining was observed at the margin of the pinguecula. The lenses were successfully worn all her waking hours on a daily-wear basis until August 1991, when she indicated a desire for extended-wear. She has been evaluated periodically for the past 2½ years and is currently a successful extended-wear patient (6 nights on, 1 off).

IV. Alternative Management Plan/Summary

Four options were available for this patient:
1. Cease contact lens wear altogether and return to spectacles.
2. Refit in RGPs once the etiology of the blurred vision in the left eye was established.
3. Referral to an ophthalmic surgeon for removal of the pinguecula and then refit her with either hydrogels or RGPs.
4. Have her wear spectacles as the primary mode of correction and the original Cibasoft daily-wear hydrogels on an occasional basis.

The disposable-lens option allowed her to continue hydrogel lens wear comfortably and successfully on an extended-wear basis. This case illustrates the importance of listening carefully to the symptomatology and matching it with the objective signs observed during the examination process.

• Case Eight: Giant Papillary Conjunctivitis

I. Subjective Data

A 29-year-old man visited our clinic after recently being transferred from New York. He had been wearing the same pair of extended-wear lenses for about 18 months, average wearing time 2 weeks between removals. He used a generic preservative saline for storage and an enzyme cleaner. A few weeks preceding this visit to our office his eyes began to feel itchy and the lenses became progressively more uncomfortable. He indicated that they tended to move around on his eyes and to have a predilection for riding under the upper lids "almost like my hard lenses did many years ago." He also noticed that there was a considerable amount of mucus floating in his eyes, which tended to blur his vision. As a result he had been removing the lenses on almost a daily basis to clean them with his surfactant. This resulted in only limited improvement, since within 20 to 30 minutes of inserting them the symptoms would reappear.

II. Objective Data

Biomicroscopy

Slit-lamp examination revealed heavily coated lenses OU that moved with every movement of the upper lid. They were coated with mucus, and lower lid retraction showed more mucus in the lower fornices. The clinical picture was typical of what might occur in a bilateral case of giant papillary conjunctivitis (GPC). Lid eversion revealed a hyperemic cobblestone appearance of the tarsal conjunctiva. The pits between the raised areas were filled with mucus, confirming the diagnosis of GPC.

Manifest refraction

OD: −3.25 DS (20/20 distance and near)
OS: −3.50 DS (20/20 distance and near)

Keratometry

OD: 40.75 @ 090; 40.50 @ 180
OS: 40.75 @ 100; 41.12 @ 010

The keratometry mires were watery and varied with the blink. However, they were free of any distortion, and their variability was most likely due to poor tear quality.

Lensometry (contact lens power)

OD: −2.50 D
OS: −2.25−2.25 D (poor mire quality resulting from heavy surface deposition)

III. Assessment/Plan

It was decided that this patient had simple myopia with GPC (grade 2+) OU. He did not have a back-up pair of spectacles. Because he was in a very high-profile position within his new company and no one had seen him wearing spectacles, he did not want to return to wearing them unless it was judged absolutely clinically essential. I explained the etiology and course of the immune process, indicating that once we removed the offending protein from its contact with the eye the lids would quiet down and he should be able to return to comfortable contact lens wear with the understanding that it would be necessary to have a cleaning regimen that assured cleanliness of the lenses. I recommended disposable lenses to be worn for as few hours as possible on a daily-wear basis for at least the first week and then requested that he remove the lenses at least once during the day to clean them thoroughly with a surfactant cleaner and rinse with preservative-free saline as an additional precaution.

When the acute phase of the GPC episode was resolved, we could cautiously return to overnight wear. A flexible wear schedule rather than extended wear was emphasized, and the patient was counseled that wearing a contact lens is not an endurance exercise to see how far we can push the envelope of safety but rather a convenient medical device to be removed more frequently than he had been doing thus far. I hoped thereby to reduce not only the possibility of a recurrence of the GPC but also the risk of a microbial infection. He agreed and stated that he had not thought of contact lenses as medical devices until now.

Contact lens prescription

Both eyes were irrigated with sterile preservative-free saline, and contact lenses with the following specifications were inserted:

		BCR	OAD	Power
OD:	Acuvue	8.8 mm	14.0 mm	−3.25 D (20/20)
OS:	Acuvue	8.8 mm	14.0 mm	−3.50 D (20/20)

Biomicroscopy

The lenses centered well, with movement patterns typical of molded lenses.

Retinoscopy over contact lenses

OU: Plano

Visual acuity with contact lenses

OD: 20/20
OS: 20/20
OU: 20/20

Subjective response

The patient reported an immediate increase in comfort although he still experienced mild itching and irritation. His vision was clear. One week later he returned for a progress evaluation. The goal of this visit was to determine whether the GPC was regressing as anticipated. He reported that the itching and mucus strands had decreased significantly but were still present. Comfortable wearing time had increased to 10 hours, and he had not found it necessary to remove the lenses for surfactant cleaning during the wearing schedule. Slit-lamp examination confirmed that the papillae were slightly smaller and there was definitely less mucus present on the tarsal conjunctiva. The old lenses were discarded and he was given a fresh sterile pair. He was monitored weekly for the next 3 weeks, and the condition continued to improved. After 4 weeks, the tarsal conjunctiva presented only minor hypertrophy and he was placed on an overnight-wear schedule. At reexamination the next day his eyes were quiet and he was instructed to remove the lenses that night for cleaning and disinfection. The wearing schedule increased to 2 nights on, with return to the office at the end of day 3.

His condition continued to show signs of improvement, so the wearing schedule was increased by 1 night each cycle (i.e., 3 nights on and 1 off for a maximum of 6 consecutive nights). Finally, he was placed on a strict 6 night/7 day maximum wear schedule (i.e., to remove more frequently if necessary but on no account to wear beyond the 6-night maximum).

There has been only one GPC recurrence in the 5 years since he first presented to our office. Fortunately, he was aware of its early warning symptoms and immediately discarded the lenses he had been wearing. He then scheduled an appointment to be examined, at which visit the presence of mild papillary hypertrophy was confirmed and he was placed on a daily-wear schedule with a 1-week discard cycle for 2 weeks. At the next follow-up visit he was returned to his flexible-wear schedule with a 1-week discard cycle. He has not experienced any further problems in the past 3 years.

IV. Alternative Management Plan/Summary

Six options were available for this patient:

1. Cease contact lens wear until signs and symptoms had resolved and then refit with a reusable extended-wear lens. However, if this were considered, it would have necessitated introducing an aggressive hygiene regimen with frequent office visits for monitoring, and he was not disposed to get so involved.
2. Same as above, with a frequent-replacement cycle (that is, more than 1 week usage). This route was not considered since he had exhibited a history of noncompliance with enzyme procedures.
3. Return to daily wear with either reusable or frequent-replacement lenses. This was also not seriously considered, for the reasons just cited.
4. Discontinue contact lens wear altogether.
5. Treat with topical steroids in conjunction with one of the contact lens treatment plans listed above. Steroid use was not considered necessary in this case.
6. Switch to RGPs. He had previously been fitted with these and had experienced discomfort.

Disposable contact lenses provide an important addition to our armamentarium in the fight to manage giant papillary conjunctivitis (GCP) created by previous modes of contact lens wear.

CLINICAL PEARL

Disposable contact lenses provide an important addition to our armamentarium in the fight to manage giant papillary conjunctivitis created by previous modes of contact lens wear.

Summary

This chapter summarizes the numerous applications for disposable lenses—some common (i.e., GPC), others not so common but nevertheless important (i.e., latent hyperopia). It is advisable to consider these lenses for any patient who desires convenience as well as the therapeutic/functional benefits that the lenses can provide.

6

Astigmatism

Thomas G. Quinn

Approximately one third of all spectacle wearers interested in contact lenses are told by their eyecare professional that they cannot wear them because they have too much astigmatism.[11] In fact, if the patient is motivated and demonstrates good ocular health and hygiene, even highly astigmatic individuals can wear contact lenses successfully. The outcome is dependent largely upon the provider's willingness to fit a toric lens. Success comes from understanding the patient's needs, knowing the mechanics of fitting, and, finally, being able to handle problems if they arise (see box). Following are examples that utilize this approach.

• Case One: Calculating Bitoric RGP Design: WTR and Oblique Cases

I. Subjective Data

A 34-year-old retail store manager expressed interest in contact lenses, chiefly for use during his hobby of sharpshooting.

II. Objective Data

Manifest refraction

OD: −1.25 −3.50 × 172 (20/20)
OS: −1.00 −2.25 × 066 (20/20)

Steps for Success in Fitting the Astigmatic Patient

Recognize the patient's needs
  Desired wearing schedule
    • All-day wear? Extended wear? Occasional wear?
  Activities (occupational and recreational)
    • Level of visual demand (e.g., accountant versus laborer)
    • Risk of lens dislocation? (e.g., football player)
    • Risk of foreign body irritation? (e.g., carpenter)
  Patient sensitivity level
    • Vision and comfort
  Refractive considerations
    • Magnitude of refractive astigmatism vs corneal toricity
    • Sphere:cylinder ratio? Axis orientation?
Select appropriate lens design
  Gas permeable
    Spherical
    Spherical base curve, toric secondary
    Back-surface toric
    Bitoric (SPE or CPE)
    Prism ballasted front-surface toric
  Soft toric
    Prism ballasted vs thin-zone stabilization
    Back-surface toric front-surface toric
    Low, medium, or high water content
    Conventional vs frequent replacement
Troubleshooting
  Analyze visual symptoms
    Constant or fluctuating?
    Immediate or late onset?
  Analyze discomfort symptoms
  Analyze lens fit
    Centration and movement
    Axis orientation
    Location and stability
  Analyze physiological response
    Slit-lamp findings
    Refractive changes?
    Keratometry changes?

Keratometry

OD: 41.00 @ 170; 44.25 @ 080 (smooth mires)
OS: 41.50 @ 065; 43.75 @ 155 (smooth mires)

The upper lid extended down over the upper limbus by 1 to 2 mm.

III. Assessment/Plan

This patient was myopic and wanted contact lenses for a visually demanding activity (sharpshooting). His visual sensitivity was assessed by using the Becherer Twist Test[3] (Table 6-1). A rotation of the best subjective cylinder result in the Phoropter by ±7° elicited a report of just noticeable blur, suggesting low tolerance for any potential axis mislocation with a toric soft lens.

It is desirable for a soft toric patient to have a spherical refractive error of at least 2 times the astigmatic error. In cases of oblique astigmatism, as in this patient's left eye, a 3:1 ratio of sphere to cylinder is preferred.[3] Furthermore, it has been shown[10,33] that the worst candidates for toric soft lenses may be low myopes with a with-the-rule astigmatism greater than the sphere power.

Rigid gas-permeable (RGP) lenses would likely offer this patient a more satisfactory visual result. Theoretically a spherical design could provide full visual correction since the corneal toricity was equal to or nearly equal the refractive astigmatism in each eye. Because this patient's upper lids extended down over the upper limbus, utilization of a *lid-attachment* fitting approach might have stabilized a spherical lens on the with-the-rule astigmatic right eye.[44] However, uneven bearing of a spherical lens on a toric cornea can have adverse mechanical effects on corneal tissue, compromising corneal physiology and leading to spectacle blur. It is unlikely that a spherical lens would have positioned in a stable fashion on the obliquely astigmatic left eye. Therefore it was decided to pursue fitting a toric rigid gas-permeable (RGP) lens to each eye.

TABLE 6-1

Becherer Twist Test (Rotate the Best Subjective Cylinder Result)

Degrees of rotation to blur	Anticipated success rate with soft torics (%)
± 20	90
± 15	90 (with 2 lenses)
± 10	70 (with 3 lenses)
± 5	Patient must accept compromised vision

Adapted from Becherer PD: *Contact Lens Update* 9(2):17-21, 1990.

Fitting

Ideally, toric RGP diagnostic lenses would be used for fitting. However, in this case appropriate trial lenses were not available so the initial pair of lenses was ordered from calculation (Fig. 6-1).[35] Keratometry and refractive findings were provided on an optical cross for organization during calculations. Because the power in the vertical meridian for the right eye was greater than 4.00 D, it was adjusted to account for the change in vertex distance. (Fig. 6-2).

A 9.5 mm lens diameter was selected to tuck the upper aspect of the lens under the upper lid. This would enhance comfort, stabilize lens positioning, and allow for a larger optical zone to reduce the potential for flare.

Base curve radius selection for the with-the-rule astigmatic right eye was made to parallel the relationship that a spherical gas-permeable lens has on a 0.75 D toric with-the-rule cornea. This relationship provided good lens translation during the blink without risking lens flexure.[18] The base curve in each meridian was flattened another 0.25 D to avoid excessive vaulting of the large lens over the cornea (Table 6-2). A decrease in minus power was made in each meridian for each dioptric unit that the corresponding base curve radius had been flattened.

The oblique orientation of the astigmatic error in the left eye required that the fitting relationship in both major meridians approximate alignment. One meridian could no longer be fitted slightly flat because the lens would then decenter along the steeper meridian. A moderate to high-Dk material was selected because the tear pump might be somewhat compromised with utilization of this saddle-fit approach. Again, to reduce vaulting with the large diameter and optical zone, a base curve radius 0.25 D flatter than measured K was selected.

Toric peripheral curves were selected to provide an even edge lift circumferentially by assessing each major meridian independently and assigning the peripheral curves customarily used with spherical lenses of the same base curve radius and diameter.[32] The final lens parameters (in millimeters) were

	BCR*	SCR	PCR	PCW	OZD
OD:	8.28/7.80	9.1/8.6	11.00/11.50 @ 0.3	9.5	7.8
OS:	8.18/7.76	9.0/8.6	11.00/11.50 @ 0.3	9.5	7.8

	BVP	CT	MATERIAL
OD:	−1.00/−3.50	0.18	Fluoroperm 60
OS:	−0.75/−3.00	0.18	Fluoroperm 60

*BCR, base curve radius; SCR, secondary curve radius; PCR, peripheral curve radius; PCW, peripheral curve width; OAD, overall diameter; OZD, optical zone diameter; BVP, back vertex power; CT, center thickness.

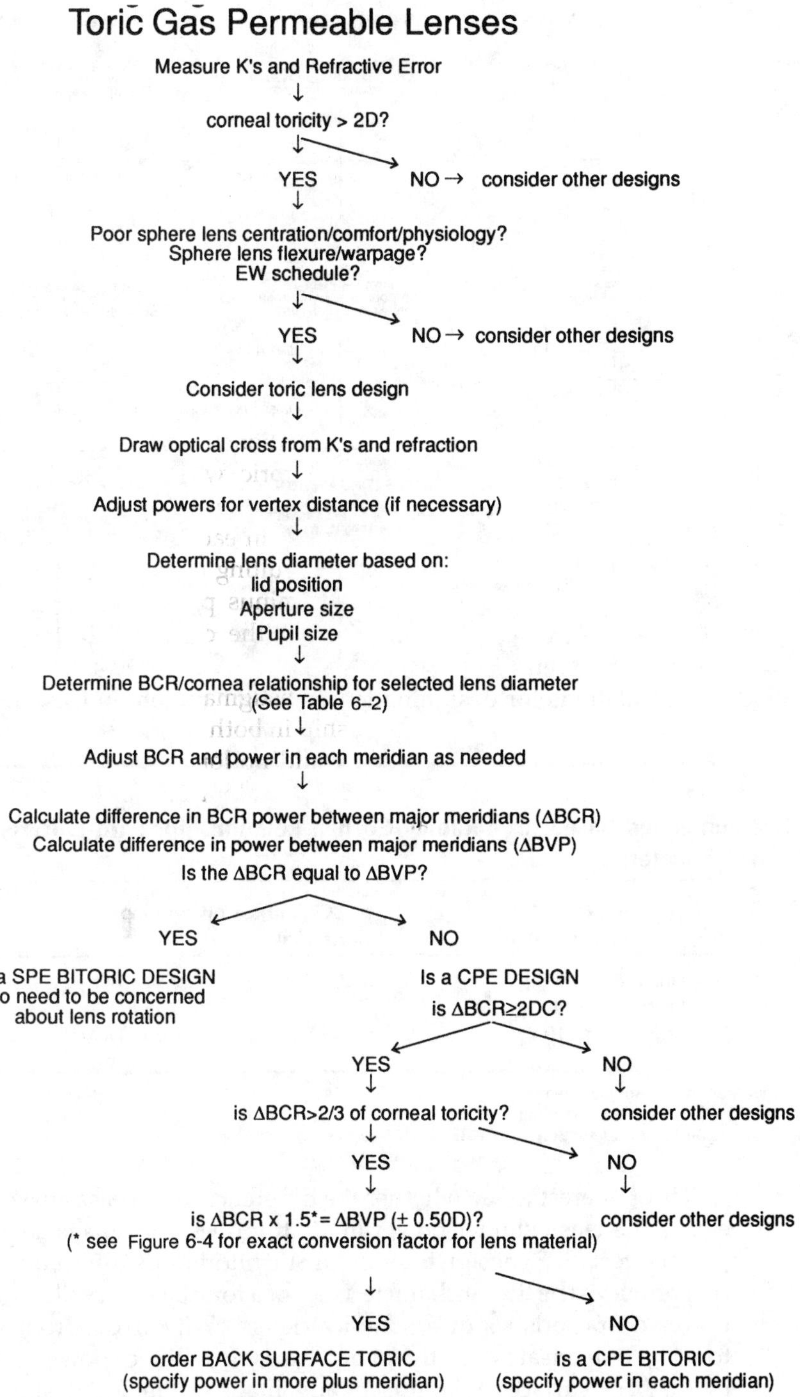

Toric Gas Permeable Lenses

Measure K's and Refractive Error
↓
corneal toricity > 2D?
↓
YES   NO → consider other designs
↓
Poor sphere lens centration/comfort/physiology?
Sphere lens flexure/warpage?
EW schedule?
↓
YES   NO → consider other designs
↓
Consider toric lens design
↓
Draw optical cross from K's and refraction
↓
Adjust powers for vertex distance (if necessary)
↓
Determine lens diameter based on:
lid position
Aperture size
Pupil size
↓
Determine BCR/cornea relationship for selected lens diameter
(See Table 6–2)
↓
Adjust BCR and power in each meridian as needed
↓
Calculate difference in BCR power between major meridians (ΔBCR)
Calculate difference in power between major meridians (ΔBVP)
Is the ΔBCR equal to ΔBVP?

YES   NO

Is a SPE BITORIC DESIGN   Is a CPE DESIGN
No need to be concerned
about lens rotation   is ΔBCR≥2DC?

YES   NO

is ΔBCR>2/3 of corneal toricity?   consider other designs
↓
YES   NO
↓   ↓
is ΔBCR x 1.5° = ΔBVP (± 0.50D)?   consider other designs
(* see Figure 6-4 for exact conversion factor for lens material)

↓

YES   NO

order BACK SURFACE TORIC   is a CPE BITORIC
(specify power in more plus meridian)   (specify power in each meridian)

FIGURE 6-1 Designing bitoric and back surface–toric gas permeable lenses by calculation. (Modified from Quinn TG: *EyeQuest* 3(4):36, 1993.)

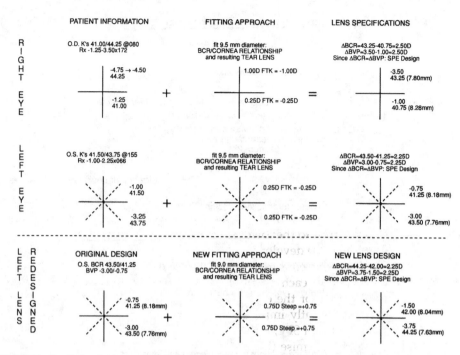

FIGURE 6-2 Calculations for designing lenses for the patient in Case 1.

TABLE 6-2

Recommended Base Curve Radius/Cornea Relationships with Different Lens Diameters

Lens diameter (mm)	BCR/Cornea relationship	
	Horizontal	Vertical;
Small (8.0 to 8.6)	0.25 STK*	0.50 FTK†
Intermediate (8.7 to 9.3)	On K	0.75 FTK
Large (9.4 to 10.2)	0.25 FTK	1.00 FTK

*STK, Steeper than the keratometric reading.
†FTK, Flatter than the keratometric reading.
Modified from Quinn TG: *EyeQuest* 3(4):36, 1993.

It is of interest to see whether the difference in the base curve power equals the lens cylinder power in air. If it does, the lens is a spherical power effect (SPE) design bitoric. An SPE bitoric lens is a unique design that provides the fitting characteristics of a toric base curve lens and the power characteristics of a spherical lens.[37] With it the front surface toricity compensates exactly for any excess of cylinder power provided by the back surface. A significant advantage of the SPE design is that the lens can rotate without inducing residual cylinder.

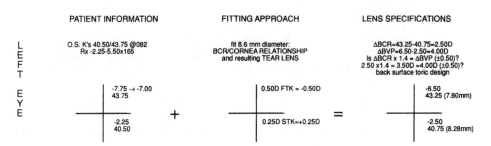

FIGURE 6-3 Calculations for designing a lens for the patient in Case 2.

Lenses were dispensed and provided excellent visual acuity. The right lens was stable and attached to the upper lid. However, the left lens dropped to the lower lid even after full adaptation was achieved, promoting the development of 3 and 9 o'clock staining and injection.[19] The lens was reordered smaller (OAD 9.0 mm, OZD 7.5 mm) and 0.75 D steeper in each meridian with −0.75 D added to the power to compensate for the change. This improved lens centration, resulting in a significantly improved corneal response. Note: The redesigned lens was still a SPE, which allowed for possible lens rotation without visual compromise (Fig. 6-2).

• Case Two: Back Surface–Toric Design; Intrapalpebral Fitting

I. Subjective Data

A 31-year-old nurse expressed interest in contact lens correction because she felt "glasses are a nuisance." She also complained of poor vision and eyestrain when wearing her glasses. She had a 10-year history of reduced vision in the left eye.

II. Objective Data

Emering spectacle correction (two years old)

OD: −1.25 −0.25 × 019 (20/50)
OS: −1.25 −0.25 × 024 (20/400)

Manifest refraction

OD: −2.25 DS (20/15)
OS: −2.25 −5.50 × 165 (20/100)

Keratometry

OD: 42.00 @ 180; 42.12 @ 090 (smooth mires)
OS: 40.50 @ 172; 43.75 @ 082 (smooth mires)

Her upper lids rested slightly above the superior limbus.

III. Assessment/Plan

This patient had a high astigmatic error in her left eye only, causing a refractive amblyopia in that eye. An increase in myopic correction for each eye, along with an astigmatic correction for the left eye, improved vision significantly.

In caring for any patient with reduced vision in one eye, it is most important that safety precautions be considered to protect the fellow "good" eye. Spectacle lens correction is generally thought to provide greater protection from ocular hazards when compared to contact lenses. However, for this patient, full spectacle correction of the large astigmatic error in the left eye was unlikely to be well tolerated because of induced prismatic effects and peripheral distortion. Thus, if spectacle correction were pursued, a compromised prescription with reduced cylindrical correction would likely have resulted in less than the maximum possible visual acuity for the left eye. In fact, this appeared to have been the approach taken by this patient's previous eyecare provider.

Full astigmatic correction was possible with contact lenses without inducing prismatic effects and meridional minification, likely resulting in better vision even than that obtained with full spectacle correction.

Since she was actively involved in detailed visual tasks and was highly motivated to pursue contact lens correction, we elected to go with an RGP lens in a toric design for the left eye. The need for proper eye safety precautions was discussed in detail and, being a nurse, she understood the importance of proper eye safety habits.

Diagnostic fitting

Because of the patient's high upper lid position relative to the superior limbus, lenses were designed for an intrapalpebral position utilizing a slightly steep base curve/cornea relationship as outlined in Table 6-2 to achieve lens centration.

An appropriate toric base curve radius lens was not available for diagnostic fitting of the left eye, so a spherical lens was selected to assess lens size and provide overrefraction data to assist in calculating lens power in a toric design. Reviewing the refractive and keratometry data I noticed that the refractive cylinder was significantly greater than the corneal toricity; therefore residual cylinder over a spherical lens would be expected. If the residual cylinder is approximately half the dioptric cylinder (0.4 for most RGPs) in the designed toric base curve and is at an axis near that of the spectacle cylinder axis (expressed in minus cylinder design), then a back-surface toric/spherical front surface design will properly correct the refractive error (Fig. 6-4). The spherical front surface allows for slight in-office adjustments in spherical power and easy front surface polishing if needed. Also the fee charged by many laboratories is less for back-surface torics than for bitoric designs. In this case 0.4 of the 2.5 D of

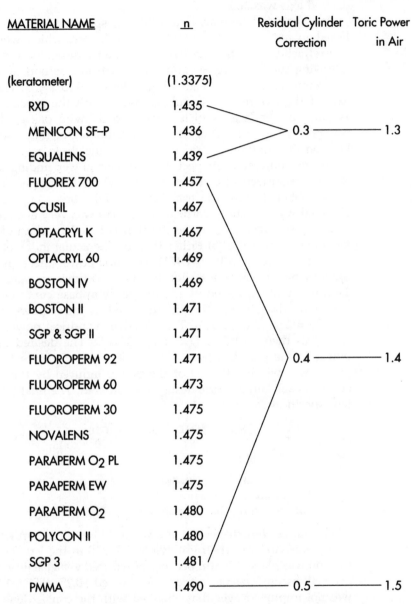

CONVERSION FACTORS to calculate:

MATERIAL NAME	n	Residual Cylinder Correction	Toric Power in Air
(keratometer)	(1.3375)		
RXD	1.435		
MENICON SF–P	1.436	0.3	1.3
EQUALENS	1.439		
FLUOREX 700	1.457		
OCUSIL	1.467		
OPTACRYL K	1.467		
OPTACRYL 60	1.469		
BOSTON IV	1.469		
BOSTON II	1.471		
SGP & SGP II	1.471		
FLUOROPERM 92	1.471	0.4	1.4
FLUOROPERM 60	1.473		
FLUOROPERM 30	1.475		
NOVALENS	1.475		
PARAPERM O_2 PL	1.475		
PARAPERM EW	1.475		
PARAPERM O_2	1.480		
POLYCON II	1.480		
SGP 3	1.481		
PMMA	1.490	0.5	1.5

FIGURE 6-4 Conversion factors for determining the power effect of toric back surfaces. *n* = index of refraction. (Modified from Quinn TG: *EyeQuest* 3(4):36, 1993.)

base curve toricity (43.25 − 40.75 = 2.50 D) would be 1.00 D and the desired axis was 165.

A polymethyl methacrylate (PMMA) spherical trial lens was selected to reduce the potential for lens flexure, which would affect overrefraction results. The lens positioned temporally and dropped following the blink. A visual acuity of 20/40 was obtained with an overrefraction showing residual cylinder of −0.75 × 135. The oblique axis of the overrefraction did not agree with the spectacle axis or keratometry findings, which agreed closely with one another. This was perhaps an artifact of the poor positioning of the spherical trial lens on an astigmatic cornea. Although the discrepancy made the overrefraction results suspect, the cylinder power finding suggested that a back surface toric design might be viable in this case. The visual acuity obtained with the trial lens (20/40) when compared to that obtained with spectacle correction (20/100) was very encouraging.

The base curve power specification is based on the index of the keratometer (n = 1.3375) rather than on the actual index of the RGP lens material (Boston II, n=1.471). The toric power effect provided by the toric base curve of a Boston II lens is 1½ times, or more precisely 1.4 times, that suggested by the difference in base curve power (Fig. 6-4). With the left lens, the difference in base curve power was 43.25 − 40.75 = 2.50 D (Fig. 6-3). The effective cylindrical power resulting from this then was 2.50 D × 1.4 = 3.50 D. The desired cylindrical power in the final lens was 6.50 − 2.50 = 4.00 D. Since the desired power was within ±0.50 D of the power induced by the toric base curve, a back surface toric design was ordered. The final (millimeter) lens specifications were

	BCR	SCR	OAD	OZD	BVP(D)	CT
OD:	8.00	9.7	8.6	7.5	−2.50	0.15
OS:	8.28/7.80	10.1/9.5	8.6	7.5	−2.50	0.15

	Material	Design
OD:	Boston II	Spherical
OS:	Boston II	Back-surface toric

The lenses were dispensed and worn. At the follow-up visit, visual acuity was 20/15 in the right eye and 20/40 in the left. The overrefraction was plano in both. Because of reduced visual acuity in the left eye, retinoscopy was performed and showed −0.25 −0.50 × 170, which was not improved over that obtained with the contact lenses. When asked about her visual performance with the lenses, the patient exclaimed, "I can't believe the difference!"

IV. Alternative Management Plan/Summary

Expanded availability in toric soft lenses provides us with the option of fitting a spherical and a toric soft lens on the right eye and left eye respectively. With an astigmatic error nearly 2.5 times the spherical error in the left eye, any slight variation in lens rotation might have compromised vision[3,10,33] although it might be well tolerated by the amblyopic eye.

• Case Three: Utilization of SPE Diagnostic Lenses (Minus Carrier Lenticular Design)

I. Subjective Data

A 16-year-old boy was fitted elsewhere approximately 3 years earlier with toric soft lenses. He wore them for a little over 2 years but reported that his vision was never satisfactory because "the lens would rotate." He was later fitted with RGP lenses. Although the vision was good, he discontinued wearing them because of discomfort experienced when they "slid down." These lenses had been returned to the fitting doctor and were not available for inspection. The patient had not worn lenses for 5 weeks before coming to my office. His desire for contact lens correction resulted primarily from the need for lens wear while playing high school basketball and for cosmetic improvement over spectacles.

II. Objective Data

Manifest refraction

OD: +6.25 −3.25 × 006   (20/20)
OS: +7.00 −3.75 × 166   (20/20−)

Keratometry

OD: 39.25 @ 010; 43.00 @ 100   (smooth mires)
OS: 38.75 @ 170; 43.00 @ 080   (smooth mires)

The upper lids covered the superior limbus.

The cover test over spectacles revealed a 2 prism diopter (Δ) esophoria at 6 M but a 4 Δ left constant esotropia at 40 cm.

III. Assessment/Plan

Because of this patient's desire to wear contact lenses while playing basketball, the first treatment option considered was a soft lens to minimize the likelihood of lens loss during participation in the sport. However, his previous experience with toric soft lenses had been unsatisfactory due to compromised vision. Consistent crisp visual correction of the right eye was of particular importance since he had a left esotropia during the performance of near tasks.

It was decided to fit him with a bitoric minus carrier lenticular RGP lens. The bitoric design would provide an optimal cornea base curve relationship to stabilize the lens fit, minimize the possible development of lens warpage, and prevent the adverse corneal effects that would likely be encountered with spherical lenses on eyes with this degree of corneal toricity. The minus carrier lenticular design allowed for a large lens diameter to utilize the upper lid and stabilize the lens position while keeping the center thickness to a minimum. Additionally, it was hoped that the large lens fitted under the upper lid would be less likely to become dislodged during participation in contact sports.

Fitting

An SPE trial lens of the following (millimeter) parameters was utilized for assessing the fit and determining lens power:

BCR	BVP (D)	OAD	OZD	CT
8.65/8.04(39.00/42.00)	Plano −3.00	9.5	7.8	0.20

A 9.5 mm diameter was selected to tuck under the lid. The base curve was almost on K horizontally and approximately 1 D flatter than K vertically (Table 6-2).

The lens was found to be large enough to ride under the upper lid and provide full optical zone coverage of the pupil without contacting the lower lid. This diameter was selected as optimal. Overrefraction results were

OD: +6.50 DS (20/20)
OS: +6.75 DS (20/20)

This power was adjusted for vertex changes from the spectacle plane to the corneal surface and added to the trial lens power (Fig. 6-5) for final lens specifications of

	BCR	SCR	Cap	ET*	JT	OAD	OZD
OD:	8.04/8.65	8.9/9.5	8.2	0.24	0.13	9.5	7.8
OS:	8.04/8.65	8.9/9.6	8.2	0.24	0.13	9.6	7.8

	BVP	CT	Material
OD:	+4.00/+7.00	0.27	Fluoroperm 60
OS:	+4.25/+7.25	0.29	Fluoroperm 60

Fluoroperm 60 was selected to provide a stable material with good oxygen permeability in this thick lens design.

Follow-up visits

After dispensing and lens wear, the patient returned for follow-up reporting that his lenses felt "better than the old (spherical) ones." He wore them "all day" with no complaints.

Visual acuity with the lenses was 20/20 OD, 20/20− OS. An overrefraction (OD plano, OS +0.25 − 0.75 × 142) did not appreciably affect vision when demonstrated through the phoropter. Both lenses consistently rode up, with the upper lids stabilizing their position. Corneal health was excellent. Although lens loss continues to be a

---

*ET, edge thickness; JT, junction thickness.

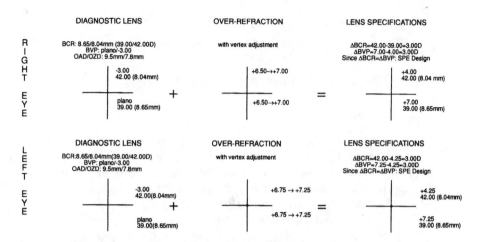

FIGURE 6-5 Calculations for designing lenses for the patient in Case 3.

potential problem with this design, no lenses have been lost after 3 years of wear.

IV. Alternative Management Plan/Summary

Reasonably clear vision could be anticipated with spherical RGP lens correction. However, the degree of corneal toricity, combined with the plus lens power needed, would probably have resulted in a low-riding lens leading to discomfort and possible corneal compromise. This might have been the mode of correction attempted by his previous provider 6 months earlier. The bitoric design provided an optimal lens cornea relationship, stabilizing the fit.

Because of his participation in active sports, a soft lens design was initially considered but rejected as described above. Had lens loss or other problems occurred with RGPs, a reassessment of toric soft lenses, beginning with the highly permeable back surface–toric designs, might have enabled me to improve performance with that design.[28]

• Case Four: Rotation of CPE Design

I. Subjective Data

A 21-year-old microbiology student expressed a desire for contact lenses, both for cosmesis and for ease of using the microscope during laboratory study. She wanted extended-wear disposable lenses for the convenience of not having to "fool with them every day."

II. Objective Data

Manifest refraction

OD: −4.00 −2.50 × 178   (20/20)
OS: −4.00 −3.25 × 002   (20/20)

Keratometry

OD: 44.00 @ 180; 46.75 @ 090   (smooth mires)
OS: 44.25 @ 180; 47.00 @ 090   (smooth mires)

The upper lid extended down over the superior limbus.

III. Assessment/Plan

This patient's significant astigmatic error obviously precluded the use of spherical disposable lenses. Although other toric soft lenses were an option, RGP lenses were selected because of their superior optical performance and greater oxygen availability during extended wear.[4,8]

Utilizing refractive and keratometric data, I designed lenses to fit near alignment in the horizontal meridian and slightly flat in the vertical meridian (Figs. 6-1 and 6-6). At dispensing, lens centration was somewhat variable because of tearing but the lenses were essentially positioned in a slightly superior location. Visual acuity was 20/30 in the right eye, 20/20 in the left.

At the follow-up visit the patient reported great improvement in comfort but complained of persistent blur in the right eye. Visual acuity again measured 20/30 in the right eye and 20/20 in the left. Overrefraction results were:

OD: +0.25 −1.25 × 034   (20/20)
OS: +0.25 DS   (20/20)

Analysis indicated that the right lens was a CPE bitoric and the left lens an SPE bitoric. Even though the base curve in the right lens met the criteria of having at least 2 D of toricity and being greater than two thirds of the corneal toricity (Fig. 6-1), the oblique orientation of the astigmatic error in the overrefraction indicated that the lens was rotating. The right lens was redesigned utilizing a saddle approach, steepening the vertical meridian to add additional toricity to the base curve and (we hoped) minimize lens rotation (Fig. 6-6).

The new right lens was dispensed and provided excellent acuity. Once she achieved successful all-day wear, the patient was permitted to sleep in her lenses and instructed to return the next morning. Good lens movement and excellent corneal response were observed. The patient is now successfully wearing her lenses and removing them at night approximately twice a week.

IV. Alternative Management Plan/Summary

Because she had a with-the-rule astigmatism and an upper lid that crossed over the superior limbus, a spherical RGP lens might have been a viable option if she had continued to have visual difficulty with the right lens. However, mechanical forces from the spherical

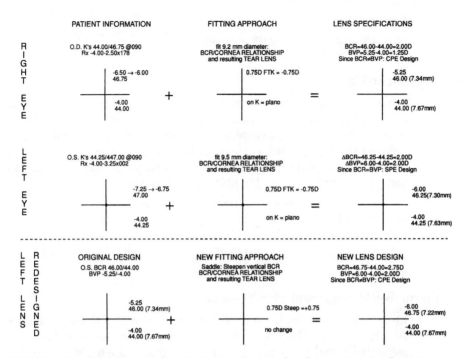

FIGURE 6-6 Calculations for designing lenses for the patient in Case 4.

lens on the toric cornea could have compromised corneal tissue and probably caused lens warpage.

Had the patient been unable to adapt to RGP lenses, a toric soft lens would have been attempted for wear on a daily-wear or, at most, a flexible wear basis (during naps and occasionally overnight).

• Case Five: Soft Spherical Versus Soft Toric with Low Astigmatism

I. Subjective Data

A 16-year-old high school football player presented to our office complaining of reduced vision with spherical daily-wear disposable lenses that he had worn successfully for 3 years.

II. Objective Data

Visual acuity with spherical soft lenses

OD: 20/25–
OS: 20/25–

Manifest refraction

OD: −3.00 −1.00 × 180 (20/20)
OS: −2.25 −0.75 × 170 (20/20)

Keratometry

OD: 45.00 @ 180; 46.25 @ 090 (smooth mires)
OS: 45.00 @ 175; 47.00 @ 085 (smooth mires)

III. Assessment/Plan

It has been shown[12] that more than 70% of low astigmats (0.75 to 1.25 D) prefer toric soft lenses over spherical lens correction. I decided to pursue toric soft lens correction for this patient. He particularly enjoyed the convenience of disposable lenses, so together we selected a monthly planned-replacement lens (55% water content, back-surface toric, prism ballasted) as his first choice (see box).

		BCR	OAD	Power
OD:	Focus toric	8.9 mm	14.5 mm	−3.00 −1.00 × 180
OS:	Focus toric	8.9 mm	14.5 mm	−2.00 −1.00 × 170

The patient is wearing the lenses successfully, with 20/20 visual acuity.

IV. Alternative Management Plan/Summary

I might have been tempted to refit this patient with a thicker spherical soft lens in an effort to mask his astigmatism, since it has been estimated[41] that spherical soft lenses can mask 20% to 70% of corneal astigmatism. However, numerous studies[6,30,40] have shown that in most cases this approach is not successful.

Another option might have been to use an RGP lens. A large steep design would help reduce the likelihood of lens loss during football. A steep fitting relationship would also promote lens flexure, desirable in this case because the corneal toricity was greater than the refractive astigmatism.[20,34] In addition, a thin design fabricated in a high-Dk material would promote lens flexure.[18]

• Case Six: Discomfort and Injection with RGPs

I. Subjective Data

A 36-year-old woman recently appointed as a university development officer complained of discomfort and injection after 6 hours of RGP lens wear. She had been taking oral antihistamines at times to control seasonal allergies. Unable to relieve her symptoms by numerous changes in solution, lens material, and lens design, I presented the option of toric soft lenses—explaining that some compromise in vision might occur relative to the clarity she had enjoyed with RGP lenses but that comfort could be significantly improved. A cylinder rotation in the Phoropter of ±15° (Table 6-1) indicated good visual tolerance of a toric soft lens.[3] She elected to pursue this option and was instructed

Toric Soft Lenses

Back surface–Toric designs

Daily wear
Accugel Custom Toric (Strieter Labs)
Biocurve Toric (California Soft Lens)
Continental Toric (Continental Contact Lens)
CSI Clarity Toric (PBH)
*Durasoft 2 Optifit Toric (Wesley Jessen)
Eclipse (Sunsoft)
Fre-Flex Toric (Optech)
Firesoft Toric (Firestone Optics)
Focus Toric (CIBA)
Horizon 55 Toric (Westcon)
Hydrocurve II 45 Toric (PBH)
Hydrocurve 3 Toric (PBH)
Hydrasoft Toric (Coast Vision)
Kontur 55 Toric Lens (Kontur Kontact Lens)
Metrosoft Toric (Metro Optics)
Multi-Flex Custom Astigmatic (Eyecare)
Ocu-Flex 53 Toric (Ocu-Ease Optical)
Opti-Fit 2 Toric (Wesley Jessen)
OPR-55 Toric (N&N Contact Lens)
*Signature Toric (PBH)
Softform II Toric (Salvatori)
Sunsoft Toric (Sunsoft)
Technicon (Great Lakes Contacts)
Torex (GBF)
Toricon (Epcon Labs)
Tresoft Toric (N&N Contact Lens)
UCL Toric 55 (United Contact Lens)
*Westhin Toric (Westcon)

Extended-Wear/Flexible-Wear Torics
*Durasoft 3 Optifit Toric (Wesley Jessen)
Eclipse (Sunsoft
Firesoft Toric FW (Firestone Optics)
Focus Toric (CIBA)
Hydrocurve II 55 Toric (PBH)
Hydrosoft Toric XW (Coast Vision)
Spectrum Toric (CIBA)
Sunsoft Toric (Sunsoft)

Tinted Torics
*Durasoft 3 Optifit Toric Colors (Wesley Jessen)

Front surface–Toric designs

†Hydromarc Toric (Vistakon)
Hydron Ultra T (Allergan)
Optima Toric (Bausch&Lomb)

*Torisoft (CIBA)

†Vistamarc Toric (Vistakon)
B&L FW Toric (Bausch&Lomb)

*Torisoft Soft Colors (CIBA)

Modified from McLaughlin R, Quinn T: *CL Spectrum* 6(1):29, 1991.
*Utilizes Thin-Zone stabilization.
†Discontinued.

to reduce her RGP lens wear by a couple of hours per day and to return after at least 1 week of no lens wear. She returned 3 weeks later.

II. Objective Data

Manifest refraction

OD: −6.00 −1.25 × 007 (20/20)
OS: −5.25 −2.25 × 167 (20/20)

Keratometry

OD: 43.25 @ 007; 44.50 @ 097   (smooth mires)
OS: 42.87 @ 170; 45.12 @ 080   (smooth mires)

Consistent results were obtained 1 week later; therefore, a refitting was performed.

III. Assessment/Plan

Ocular surface drying was thought to have played some role in this patient's problems with RGP lenses. Studies[2] have shown that thicker soft lenses can reduce dehydration effects during wear, so a back surface–toric prism-ballasted design (55% water content) was selected for this patient.

Diagnostic lenses

	BCR	OAD	Power
OD:	Std	14.5 mm	−1.75 −1.25 × 175
OS:	Std	14.5 mm	−2.00 −1.75 × 180

After settling, the lenses were observed to move and center well. The right lens did not rotate, and the left lens rotated 10° nasally. When a lens was manually displaced, it returned to the same location, indicating good stability of rotation.[9] Lenses were ordered with an axis adjustment made in the left lens to account for the observed rotation. Vertex adjustments reduced the sphere power by 0.50 D but did not significantly affect cylinder power. However, a slight reduction in cylinder power was made in anticipation of incomplete flexure of the thick prism-ballasted lenses.[45]

Ordered lenses

	BCR	OAD	Power
OD:	Std	14.5 mm	−5.75 −1.00 × 005
OS:	Std	14.5 mm	−4.75 −2.00 × 180

At dispensing, neither lens rotated significantly. The patient was able to achieve visual acuity of 20/20 and 20/25 in the right and left eyes. One week later she returned reporting excellent comfort but variable vision. Visual acuity was 20/25 and 20/30. The right lens was rotating 10° nasal and the left was now rotating 10° temporal!

It was obvious that, even though the diagnostic lenses were stable, the rotational stability of the prescription lenses was poor. This was probably due to increased interaction between the lids and the thicker edge of the higher-minus prescription lenses. Toric soft lens orientation is least predictable when correcting with-the-rule refractive errors,[17,33,42] probably because of interaction between the upper lid and the thicker edge associated with the more minus vertical meridian.[21] In an effort to reduce this effect many toric lenses available today have the cylinder power confined to the optical zone, providing a more even edge thickness around the circumference of the lens.[1,3]

IV. Alternative Management Plan/Summary

A change in base curve radius or diameter might have improved rotational stability. An excessively loose lens would rotate in a haphazard fashion, as was observed here. Conversely, a lens that was too steep might "lock" at an off-axis location or slowly creep in a given direction.[24] No other base curve radius was available in the unsuccessful design used in this case. The patient was subsequently fitted with another back surface–toric prism-ballasted design in a low–water content material (CSI Toric) and had good success.

• Case Seven: Prism vs Thin Zones; Front-Surface vs Back-Surface Soft Toric

I. Subjective Data

A 22-year-old mother with longstanding amblyopia in the right eye had successfully worn a 58% water–content prism-ballasted front surface toric soft lens (Vistamarc Toric) for 7 years. Her current lenses were 22 months old and in need of replacement. However, the lens she had worn successfully for so many years was no longer available, necessitating a refit into a new lens design.

II. Objective Data

Retinoscopy

OD: +3.50 –1.00 × 095 (20/400)
OS: +3.50 –1.25 × 098 (20/25)

Manifest refraction

OD: Unattainable
OS: +3.00 –1.00 × 170 (20/20)

Keratometry

OD: 41.75 @ 180; 42.75 @ 090 (smooth mires)
OS: 42.62 @ 180; 42.75 @ 090 (smooth mires)

Cover test

6 M: 6 exo with 8 right hypertropia
40 cm: 8 exo with 8 right hypertropia

Biomicroscopy

No evidence of corneal edema or staining was observed.

III. Assessment/Plan

Because of the long-term success this patient had experienced with toric soft lenses, it was decided to stay with this approach. She had a significant hyperopic refractive error, so a lens of moderate to high water content was chosen to aid oxygen transmissibility. Although a prism-ballasted design would increase thickness and reduce oxygen transmissibility, she had worn such a design successfully for many years. Therefore, she was refitted into a 55% water content prism-ballasted back surface–toric lens with the following parameters:

	BCR	OAD	BVP
OD:	8.6 mm	14.5 mm	+3.25 −0.75 × 095
OS:	8.6 mm	14.5 mm	+3.25 −0.75 × 095

At dispensing and follow-up visits she reported good comfort with the new lenses and achieved 20/20 vision in the left eye. However, she returned 5 months later complaining of injection and discomfort after 4 to 5 hours of wear. She had worn the lenses for 2 hours before this visit. She denied taking any medication and continued to use the same chemical care system she had been using successfully for 4 years. Further discussion revealed that she had experienced discomfort late in the day with the new lenses from the very start but had assumed it was part of adaptation.

Visual acuity with the left lens was 20/25 with an insignificant overrefraction. The lenses appeared to be clean and to move well on the eye. Punctate staining of the inferior cornea was evident along with 2+ conjunctival injection. Keratometry findings were

OD: 41.87 @ 162; 42.25 @ 072   (smooth mires)
OS: 42.75 @ 037; 42.12 @ 127   (smooth mires)

It was possible that inferior corneal staining could have been caused by dryness. However, this was unlikely since she had not experienced the problem with her other lenses and the thickness of a prismatic soft lens is generally helpful in reducing dryness problems.[2]

Although no corneal striae were evident, it was concluded that her symptoms were due to hypoxia resulting from the lower water content and thicker design (prism increased from 1.12 to 1.5 Δ) of the new lenses.

She was refitted with a 55% water–content back surface–toric lens utilizing thin zones for stabilization rather than prism (Durasoft 3

Optifit Toric). The goal was to reduce lens thickness to increase oxygen supply through the lens. The patient continues to wear this design, with excellent comfort, vision, and physiological response.

IV. Alternative Management Plan/Summary

Although conventional wisdom suggests that a front surface–toric (the design of this patient's original Vistamarc Toric lenses) would have been preferable for this patient's nearly spherical cornea, a back surface–toric design (Durasoft 3 Optifit Toric) is performing quite well. It is also commonly thought[29] that back-surface torics perform better on highly toric corneas. Both front- and back-surface torics have proven effective in correcting astigmatic errors of 2 D or less.[16,22,23,43] Lenses of higher toricity (see box) have been available only in back surface–toric designs, so this controversy has not been an issue in those power ranges. That may change with the introduction of higher cylinder powers in front surface toric designs. It has been suggested[31] that practitioners have both a front surface–toric and a back surface–toric design available in their offices so the other option will be available if one is not successful.

Toric soft lenses have been found to demonstrate the greatest rotational stability when correcting against-the-rule astigmatic errors.[17,33,36,42] This is thought to be due to the fact that the meridian with the higher minus power, and therefore the thicker edge, lies in the horizontal meridian parallel to the lids. Thus the lids blink over the thin superior and inferior lens edges, minimizing lid/lens interaction and preventing potential destabilizing effects.[21] Prism-ballasted designs commonly have the lower aspect of the lens thinned to reduce potentially disruptive lower lid forces and improve comfort. Lenses utilizing a double thin zone stabilization design (see box) particularly complement the thickness distribution in an axis 090 lens.[17]

If this patient had continued to suffer from hypoxia, an RGP might have been attempted, since it would provide greater levels of oxygen to the eye than a soft lens design would.[8] Keratometry findings indicated that the left cornea was nearly spherical so no tear lens would have been created to correct the astigmatic error. (It is advisable to confirm this with a spherical trial lens.) If residual astigmatism had been found, a front surface–toric prism–ballasted design would have been needed.[7]

Front surface–toric prism–ballasted RGP lenses tend to position low so should generally be fitted using a large diameter to reduce flare. The amount of prism needed increases with higher minus powers to counteract the increased thickness of the superior aspect of the lens. A prism of 0.75 to 2.5 $\triangle$ is generally prescribed. Anticipate the base to rotate approximately 10° nasally because of lid forces.[5] It has been suggested[25] that rotational characteristics may vary with changes in RGP lens materials.

• Case Eight: Irregular Draping Effects on Vision; Overrefraction Analysis

I. Subjective Data

A 29-year-old pressman at the local newspaper had successfully worn RGP lenses for 3 years but had discontinued lens wear 6 months earlier, expressing interest in soft contact lens correction for better comfort.

II. Objective Data

Manifest refraction

OD: +2.50 −1.25 × 022   (20/20)
OS: +0.75 −0.75 × 003   (20/20)

Keratometry

OD: 42.12 @ 020; 43.50 @ 110   (smooth mires)
OS: 43.12 @ 180; 43.75 @ 090   (smooth mires)

II. Assessment/Plan

It was suggested to the patient that he bring his RGP lenses in for inspection to see whether polishing or refitting could improve their comfort. However, he was quite insistent and motivated to attempt soft lens wear, so this was pursued.

Because of hyperopia in the right eye, a lens of medium to high water content was selected to reduce the potential for corneal hypoxic stress. Appropriate diagnostic lenses were not available so lenses were empirically fitted in accordance with the manufacturer's recommendations based on keratometry and refractive data. This has been shown[27,33,39] to be a valid approach.

Ordered lenses

		BCR	OAD
OD:	Hydrasoft toric	8.9 mm	15.0 mm
OS:	Hydrasoft toric	8.9 mm	15.0 mm

	Desired power	Actual power
OD:	+3.00 −1.25 × 022	+3.00 −1.25 × 020
OS:	+1.00 −0.75 × 003	+1.00 −1.00 × 003

At dispensing, the lenses appeared to move somewhat excessively and the vision was variable. This persisted when the patient returned 1 week later complaining that the lenses "slopped around a lot" resulting in discomfort and variable vision. Visual acuity was 20/40 OD and 20/25 OS. Attempts at overrefraction did not improve vision. The lenses had been worn for 12 hours before the visit yet demonstrated excessive movement. Both rotated in a haphazard fashion. Although keratometry findings were within the range expected to perform well with this base curve radius, clinical observations indicated that a steeper base curve radius was needed; thus the same power was ordered in an 8.6 mm base curve radius.

The patient found the steeper lenses to be much more comfortable. Vision in the left eye was significantly improved, yet he complained of persistent blur with the right lens. Again, refraction over the right lens did not significantly or consistently improve vision. He volunteered that vision with the right lens would clear after a hard blink. Viewing through an ophthalmoscope at arm's length from the patient demonstrated a clear red reflex immediately after the blink followed seconds later by a gray distortion.

Proper draping of the lens over the cornea is important not only physiologically but also visually. Aside from its effects on stability of rotation (Case 6), an improper fitting relationship can cause irregular lens flexure. A patient wearing an excessively steep-fitting lens may report improved vision immediately after the blink, as in this case. It is essential not to be misled by a coated lens surface, which may result in similar symptoms. Observation of the red reflex or keratometry mires over the lens, as well as direct observation of the cleanliness of the lens, can be used to distinguish between these phenomena.[41] In addition, a properly fitted back surface–toric lens, like the one used here, should have a nearly spherical overkeratometry measurement.[14]

If improper flexure is observed and adjustment of the base curve radius does not solve the problem, modification of lens thickness may be helpful.[14] This approach made sense to me in light of the fact that the thinner left lens was providing excellent vision. Therefore an 8.9 mm lens was reordered for the right eye in the thinner Hydrosoft Toric XW design.

After 1 week of wearing the thinner right lens the patient returned indicating that the right lens was still somewhat blurred; however, vision did not appear to fluctuate with blinking. Visual acuity was 20/30 but improved to a stable 20/20 with an overrefraction of −0.25 −0.50 × 055. The lens moved and centered well with a consistent 5° nasal rotation of the prism base.

Although some general guidelines for power changes indicated by the overrefraction may be followed[38] (see box), combining the crossed cylinders of the lens and the overrefraction gives more definitive data. This can be performed using lenses in a trial frame and measuring the resultant power with a lensometer or by computer calculation. Although questioned by some,[26] the manufacturer recommends the observed lens rotation not be factored into the computer calculation.[13,15] This method suggested a new lens power of +2.75 −1.25 × 027. The resultant cylinder axis made sense with the observed rotation of the lens so a new lens was ordered in this power. With this lens the patient has achieved clear and consistent 20/20 vision.

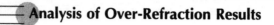

Analysis of Over-Refraction Results

Overrefraction results	Lens adjustment
OR axis = Refraction axis	Increase lens cylinder power
OR axis = 90 degrees away	Decrease lens cylinder power
OR sphere/cylinder* at oblique axis	Adjust axis

	Axis Mislocation
OR cylinder = Lens cylinder power	Lens is 30° off axis
OR cylinder = One third lens cylinder power	Lens is 10° off axis

*The cylinder component will be double the sphere component.
Modified from McLaughlin R, Quinn T: *CL Spectrum* 6(1):29-31, 1991.

Summary

The contact lens alternatives for correcting astigmatism presented in this chapter are very important for appropriate use in contact lens practice. Both rigid and soft toric lens designs are indicated in a significant percentage of interested patients. To use other nonastigmatic correcting options would not produce optimum visual acuity and might, in some cases, compromise the lens/cornea fitting relationship.

Bibliography

1. Ames K, Erickson P, Medici L: Factors influencing hydrogel toric lens rotation, *Int Contact Lens Clin* 16(7,8):221, 1989.
2. Andrasko GA, Schoessler JP: The effect of humidity on the dehydration of soft contact lenses in the eye, *Int Contact Lens Clin* 17(5):210-212, 1980.
3. Becherer PD: Soft torics, a viable modality, *Contact Lens Update* 9(2):17-21, 1990.
4. Bennett ES, Ghormley NR: Rigid extended wear: an overview, *Int Contact Lens Clin* 14(8):319-331, 1987.
5. Bergmanson J: Front toric rigid contact lens design: an easy solution to a common problem, *Contact Lens J* 16(5):105, 1988.
6. Bernstein PR, Gundel RE, Rosen JS: Masking corneal toricity with hydrogels: does it work? *Int Contact Lens Clin* 18(3-4):67-70, 1991.
7. Bier N, Lowther GE: *Contact lens correction*, Boston, 1979, Butterworth.
8. Brennan NA, Efron N, Holden BA: Further developments in the RGP Dk controversy, *Int Eyecare* 2(10):508-509, 1986.
9. Buckley DD: Torics: potential abounds, *Contact Lens Spectrum* 8(2):30, 1993.
10. Castellano CF, et al: Rotational characteristics and stability of soft toric lenses, *J Am Optom Assoc* 61(3):167-170, 1990.
11. Contact Lens Council Annual meeting, 1991.

PLATE 1 Steep fitting relationship with a spherical base curve rigid gas-permeable (RGP) lens on a 3 D with-the-rule cornea. Note the double D appearance of the steep fit on a with-the-rule astigmatic cornea.

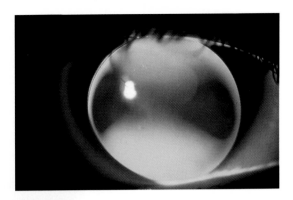

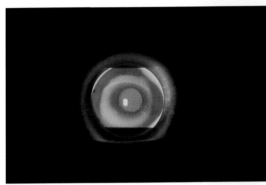

PLATE 2 Bulls-eye appearance with peripheral staining denoting overly large lens diameter in a vascularized limbal keratitis patient.

PLATE 3 Cornea after removal of a rigid gas-permeable (RGP) lens that had become adherent. Note the "strand of pearls" caused by bubbles trapped under the lens edge.

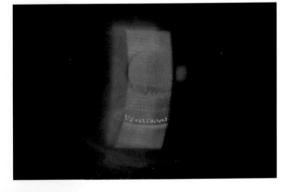

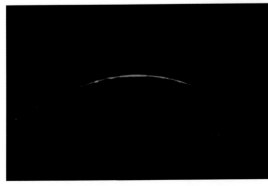

PLATE 4 Tricurve lens, posterior surface profile.

PLATE 5 Aspheric lens, posterior surface profile.

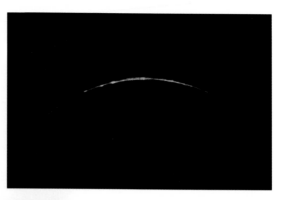

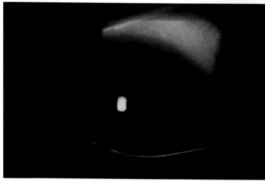

PLATE 6 Preservative reaction. (Courtesy Randy McLaughlin, M.S., O.D.)

PLATE 7 Mucoprotein-coated rigid lens.

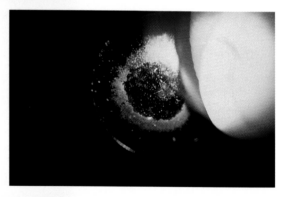

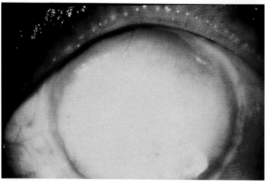

PLATE 8 *Pseudomonas* ulcer from "topping off." (Courtesy Larry J. Davis, O.D.)

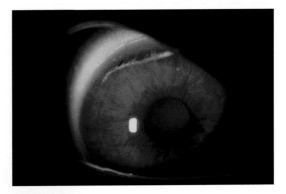

PLATE 9 Epithelial splitting.

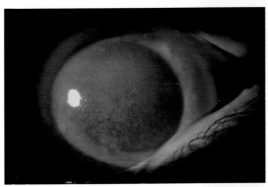

PLATE 10 Preservative hypersensitivity reaction.

PLATE 11 A properly positioned Lifestyle Hi-Rider multifocal rigid lens.

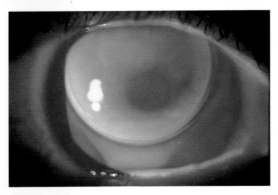

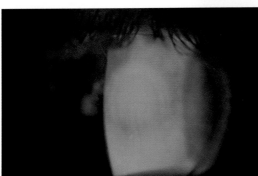

PLATE 12 The center/distance aspheric Multisite multifocal rigid lens.

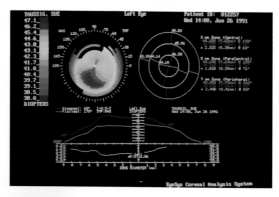

PLATE 13 Computerized videokeratography (EyeSys Laboratories, Houston, Texas) of the left cornea, Case One.

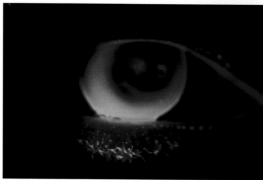

PLATE 14 Flat-fitting keratoconus contact lens. Notice the scarring in the central cornea.

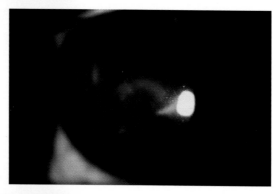

PLATE 15 Superficial central scarring, which may be exacerbated by a rigid contact lens that fits excessively flat.

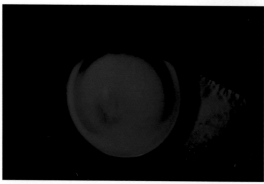

PLATE 16 Dye pattern after refitting Case Three. A "three-point touch" fitting relationship is demonstrated.

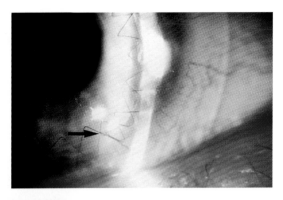

PLATE 17 Neovascularization along suture bites associated with a tight-fitting soft contact lens after penetrating keratoplasty.

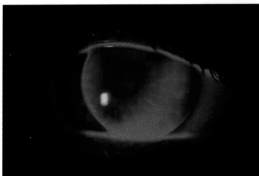

PLATE 18 Fitting relationship of a rigid gas-permeable (RGP) contact lens after penetrating keratoplasty, Case Four.

PLATE 19 Placido's disc on a graft that has decentered slightly. Irregular astigmatism is often associated with a decentered graft.

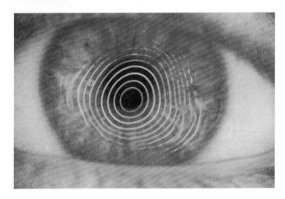

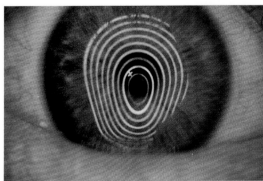

PLATE 20 Placido's disc in pellucid degeneration. Notice the marked steepening and high astigmatism inferior to the visual axis. (Courtesy Patrick J. Caroline, C.O.T., F.A.A.O., Portland, Ore.)

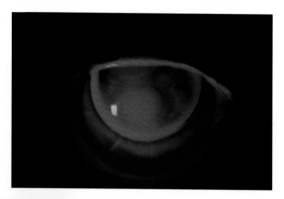

PLATE 21 Dye pattern following radial keratotomy. Notice the central clearance/fitting relationship.

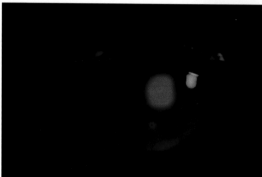

PLATE 22 Corneal epithelial abrasion induced by an RGP lens edge or fingernail.

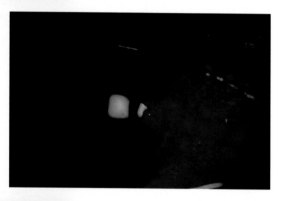

PLATE 23 Corneal infiltrate associated with daily-wear disposable soft contact lenses.

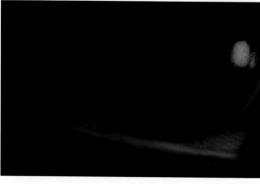

PLATE 24 A, Inferiorly decentered RGP lens rubbing against an immunologically active limbus.

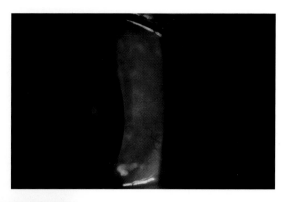

PLATE 24 B, Peripheral superficial vascularization of the cornea induced by RGP decentration.

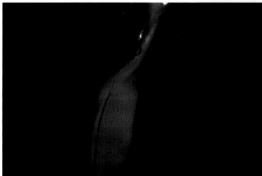

PLATE 25 A, An 8.8 mm lenticular RGP lens encroaching on the margin of a filtering bleb.

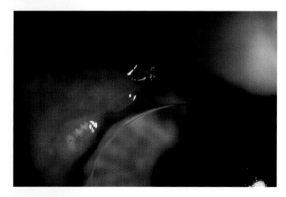

PLATE 25 B, An 8.4 mm single-cut RGP lens moving freely away from the bleb.

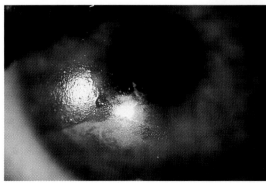

PLATE 26 Anterior surface plaque on a hydrogel lens.

PLATE 27 A, Subtle difficult-to-see vertical arclike fracture of a tangent street bifocal lens (indirect illumination).

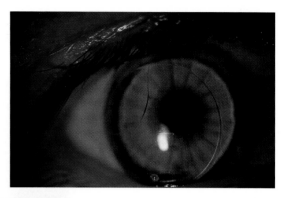

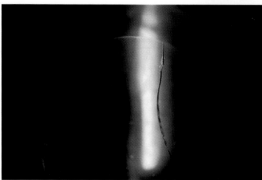

PLATE 27 B, Easier-to-visualize lens fracture (indirect retroillumination).

PLATE 28 A, Contracted hydrogel lens edge slightly indenting a localized area of the conjunctiva.

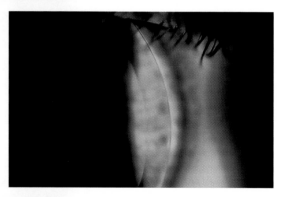

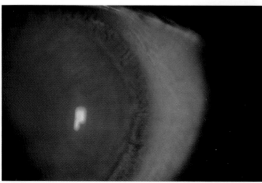

PLATE 28 B, Intralimbal radial pattern staining of the cornea after lens removal and irrigation. Notice also the lingering conjunctival stain.

12. Dabkowski JA, Roach MP, Begley CG: Soft toric versus spherical contact lenses in myopes with low astigmatism, *Int Contact Lens Clin* 19(11,12):252-255, 1992.

13. Dishman A, et al: Using crossed cylinders resolution to solve toric soft lens acuity problems, *Contact Lens Spectrum* 7(4):29-35, 1992.

14. Eiden SB: Precision management of high astigmats with toric hydrogel contact lenses, *Contact Lens Spectrum* 7(6):43-48, 1992.

15. Geller J: Consultant's corner, *Keeping In Contact (CoastVision Newsletter)*, October 1992.

16. Goldsmith WA, Steel S: Rotational characteristics of toric contact lenses, *Int Contact Lens Clin* 18(11-12):227-229, 1991.

17. Gundel R: Effect of cylinder axis on rotation for a double thin zone design toric hydrogel, *Int Contact Lens Clin* 16(5):141-151, 1989.

18. Harris MG, Chu CS: The effect of contact lens thickness and corneal toricity on flexure and residual astigmatism, *Am J Optom Arch Am Acad Optom* 49:304-307, 1972.

19. Henry VA, Bennett ES, Forrest JF: Clinical investigation of the Paraperm EW rigid gas permeable contact lens, *Am J Optom Physiol Opt* 64(5):313-320, 1987.

20. Herman JP: Flexure of rigid contact lenses on toric corneas as a function of base curve fitting relationship, *J Am Optom Assoc* 54(3):209-213, 1983.

21. Holden BA: The principles and practice of correcting astigmatism with soft contact lenses, *Aust J Optom* 58:279-299, 1975.

22. Jurkus JM, Furman DW, Colip MK: Stability characteristics of toric soft lenses, *Int Contact Lens Clin* 20(3,4):65-68, 1993.

23. Jurkus JM, Gindorf M, Hassinger M: A comparison of rotational characteristics of front and back surface toric hydrogel lenses, *Optom Month*, pp 534-539, October 1983.

24. Jurkus J, et al: The effect of fit and parameter changes on soft lens rotation, *Am J Optom Physiol Opt* 56(12): 734-736, 1979.

25. Kasti P, Johnson W: Fluoroperm: front toric fitting, *CLAO J* 16(1):53, 1990.

26. Lawson JL: Toric lens rotation and crossed-cylinder resolution, *Contact Lens Spectrum* 8(8):13-14, 1993.

27. Lieblein JS, Wells MM: To trial fit torics or not, *Contact Lens Spectrum* 6(4):35-37, 1991.

28. Maltzman BA: Astigmatic corneas: an approach to the difficult soft lens fit, *Contact Lens Update* 9(1):13-16, 1990.

29. Maltzman BA, Rengel A: Soft toric lenses: correcting cylinder greater than sphere, *CLAO J* 15(3):196-198, 1989.

30. McCarey BE, Amos CF, Taub LR: Surface topography of soft contact lenses for neutralizing corneal astigmatism, *CLAO J* 19(2):114-120, 1993.

31. McLaughlin R, Quinn T: RGP versus soft torics: which is better? *Contact Lens Spectrum* 6(1):29-31, 1991.

32. Michaud L, Sevigny J: Astigmatism revisited: a case report, *Int Contact Lens Clin* 19(9&10):215-220, 1992.

33. Myers RI, Jones DH: Can soft toric lenses be empirically fitted? *Contact Lens Spectrum* 5(3):41-45, 1990.

34. Pole JJ: The effect of the base curve on the flexure of Polycon lenses, *Int Contact Lens Clin* 10(1):49-52, 1983.

35. Quinn TG: Tackling RGP Torics, *EyeQuest* 3(4):36-50, 1993.

36. Quinn TG: Proven toric lens fitting strategies, *Contact Lens Spectrum* 9(3):22-26, 1994.

37. Sarver MD, Kame RT, Williams CE: A bitoric gas permeable hard contact lens with spherical power effect, *J Am Optom Assoc* 56(3):184-189, 1985.

38. Snyder C: A review and discussion of crossed cylinder effects and overrefractions with soft toric lenses, *Int Contact Lens Clin* 16(4):113-117, 1989.

39. Snyder C, Bowling EL: Diagnostic versus empirical fitting with the Eclipse Toric soft lens, *Contact Lens Spectrum* 5(12):29-34, 1990.

40. Snyder C, Talley D: Masking astigmatism with selected spherical soft contact lenses, *J Am Optom Assoc* 60(10):728-731, 1989.

41. Stein H, Slatt B: *Fitting guide for rigid and soft contact lenses,* St Louis, 1984, Mosby.

42. Tomlinson A, Bibby MM: Lid interaction and toric soft lens axis location, *Am J Optom Physiol Opt* 59(3):228-233, 1982.

43. Tomlinson A, Chang F, Hitchcock J: A comparison of the stability of front and back surface toric soft lenses, *Int Eyecare* 2(4):218-222, 1986.

44. Weissman BA: *Contact lens primer: a manual,* Philadelphia, 1984, Lea & Febiger.

45. Weissman BA: Theoretical optics of toric hydrogel contact lenses, *Am J Optom Physiol Opt* 63(7):536-538, 1986.

7

Presbyopia

Melvin J. Remba

Contact lens fitting to the presbyopic eye has been, and is still today, probably one of the most challenging and yet rewarding professional experiences of the contact lens clinician. The presbyopic eye not only is optically different from the younger eye (due to the gradual reduction and eventual loss of accommodation) but is also anatomically and physiologically changing with age. These changes, which affect the acceptance and performance of contact lenses, include the reduction of lid tonicity, tear quality and volume, and corneal sensitivity and, perhaps more important, a loss of luminance to the retina as changes in the internal ocular media progress normally with aging.

Perhaps the most difficult aspect(s) of contact lens fitting to the patient who requires different optical powers for clear distance and near vision is (are) the optical construction and lens function. The key is placing the proper lens power (of its two or more power zones) before the visual axis while the subject is gazing at the object of regard, with minimal interference and competition from the other lens power zones. Translating rigid gas-permeable (RGP) lenses, which are made with prism ballast for nonrotation and are constructed with add segments in the lower region, utilizes the *alternating-vision* mechanism to attain this desired visual function as the gaze is raised and lowered. Unfortunately, hydrogel lenses of similar design have not been as successful, because their inherent size and vertical movement dynamics do not allow for adequate lens translation and recovery while shifting gaze.

Concentric, aspheric (progressive-add) and diffractive hydrogel lenses have been developed, some having evolved from the early technologies of rigid corneal lenses. They function using the *simultaneous-vision* mechanism, which means that the two (or more) primary power zones are positioned within the pupillary aperture and the patient "selects" from the multiple, often superimposed, images that form on the retina. This is a "blur interpretative" cortical process that is learned and varies among individuals. It requires an adaptation period that clinicians observe in multifocal fitting and varies in length from patient to patient.

Simultaneous-vision lenses depend not on controlled zone movement and positioning but on centration, and the diameters of the near/distance zones or the eccentricity of the aspheric geometry are critical issues in their design and manufacture. Recent improvements in the manufacturing of aspherical multifocal RGP lenses are converting these to viable alternatives for presbyopic contact lens correction as well.

The oldest and still most commonly used fitting technique for presbyopia is monovision, wherein usually the sighting dominant eye is corrected with a distance power lens. Successful adaptation to monovision is thought to occur by "blur suppression" of the competing retinal image from the contralateral eye. In view of the obvious binocular compromises, the success rate for this fitting modality is remarkably high.

There are many types and brands of rigid and soft multifocal lenses, each with its own biases of clear vision ranges, advantages, and disadvantages, and most involve some visual compromise by the lens user. Clinicians are sorting out the optical characteristics of these designs and learning to match the best type of lens to the specific patient's ocular characteristics and occupational needs. It is also evident, from the case reports that follow, that, in addition to familiarity with lens design and lens function, both patience and skill are required to fit multifocal lenses successfully.

Ten respected clinicians, each experienced in presbyopic contact lens management, have contributed case reports in this chapter. The reports pertain to a wide spectrum of fitting alternatives and reflect the unique style and perhaps particular preferences of the fitter, and yet all recount continuing success with multifocal lenses, while acknowledging that success with hydrogel bifocals is still less than desired.

I wish now to acknowledge these contributors: Drs. Robert A. Koetting, Joe B. Goldberg, Shahane T. Kirman, Bruce A. Bridgewater, Jack J. Yager, Kenji Hamada, Douglas Becherer, David Hansen, Jerome Lieblein, and Joseph Vehige.

• Case One: Monovision

I. Subjective Data

A 50-year-old woman reported to our office with a desire to eliminate the inconvenience of wearing reading glasses. She had been using a computer and reading directories, correspondences, and contracts in her position in real estate sales. On the advice of her previous doctor, she was wearing +1.50 D "high-fashion" plastic readers; but she also owned several other pairs of glasses of unknown prescription. Her general health appeared to be good, and she was not taking any medications.

Visual acuity unaided

OD: 20/20
OS: 20/20
OU: 20/20

II. Objective Data

Manifest refraction

OD: +0.25 − 0.50 × 175 (20/20+)
OS: +0.25 − 0.25 × 010 (20/20+)

Autokeratometry

OD: 43.00 @ 180; 43.37 @ 090 (smooth mires)
       Shape +0.27
OS: 42.87 @ 010; 43.25 @ 100 (smooth mires)
       Shape +0.33

Diagnosis - Emmetropia with early presbyopia.

Biomicroscopy/anatomical measurements

Tear B.U.T. (break-up time)	15 sec
Blink rate	16/min
Palpebral fissure	Medium
Low lid position	At limbus
V.I.D. (visible iris diameter)	11.2 mm
Pupil	OD 3.5 mm, OS 3.5 mm
Lid tension	Normal OU
Fusion and binocularity	Normal

III. Assessment/Plan

Several options were available for this patient. It was decided to select a single-vision spherical hydrogel lens on one eye only (monovision), recognizing the patient's preference for no distance correction and to be consistent with her occupation and social visual requirements while causing minimum annoyance and physical discomfort. In addition, it was the least complex alternative.

Examination procedure

Although it was anticipated that the patient would wear only one hydrogel lens, the examination included RGP and hydrogel lenses on both eyes. Use of rigid lenses allowed evaluation of fluorescein patterns and overrefraction to verify keratometric measurements. Furthermore, patient reaction to both modalities could be studied and recorded. Even though a lens might be prescribed for one eye at first, bilateral observations would be useful if the second eye was fitted at a later date.

A near lens would preferably, and usually, be worn on the non-dominant eye, which would leave the other eye available for sighting (as with a camera) and has generally proven to be most satisfactory. The final choice involved holding a trial lens (in this case +1.75 D) before the right eye, with the left focused for distance, while instructing the patient to shift view from a reading card to the projected chart. This was repeated with the near lens before the left eye. After several attempts it became evident with a reading lens before the left eye interfered least with distance viewing while providing adequate correction for reading.

A daily-wear 38% water content hydroxyethyl methacrylate (HEMA) 8.7 mm BCR, 14.0 mm OAD +1.75 D lens (Optima) was selected from inventory for the left eye. Movement of the lens with the blink was 0.5 mm and near acuity was J1 at 16 inches in the right eye.

Note: Contrary to a philosophy expressed by some clinicians, I arbitrarily prescribe the full near correction or even a +0.25 D add overcorrection for near while undercorrecting distance vision if possible. This assures quicker adaptation, because the distance correction cannot be used for reading, or vice versa, and there is a greater out-of-focus interval, with less competition between the eyes.[1]

CLINICAL PEARL

Contrary to a philosophy expressed by some clinicians, I arbitrarily prescribe the full near correction or even a +0.25 D add overcorrection for near while undercorrecting distance vision if possible. This assures quicker adaptation, because the distance correction cannot be used for reading, or vice versa, and there is a greater out-of-focus interval, with less competition between the eyes.[1]

The patient was permitted a half-hour adaptation time in the office and then asked directly: "Do you feel you could drive safely wearing this lens for a period of 6 weeks?" Also, "Do you feel you could work efficiently for 6 to 8 weeks with no other lens correction?" These two questions were followed by the advice, "If you feel you could get along with your vision as it is now for 6 to 8 weeks, I can assure you that you will adapt to the lenses without difficulty. On the other hand, if you have any serious concern that you won't be able to use them all day, every day, for that length of time, we had better take some other approach to solving your problem."

Dispensing

OD: 20/20   (no lens)
OS: 20/40-   (with lens)

Recognizing that most presbyopes often have a fear of handling lenses, our instructor called her the day after the training/delivery session to confirm that she had not encountered any difficulty. Some clumsiness was reported followed by assurance that all was well.

Return schedule: 1 week, 1 month, and every 6 months thereafter
Wearing time: 12 hours maximum per day for the first week
and full time after that

IV. Alternative Management Plan/Summary

Several other options could be considered for this patient:
1. Translating bifocal RGP or hydrogel lenses. She was presently satisfied with her distance vision and most likely would be annoyed by a near-plano distance contact lens of this type.
2. Simultaneous-vision bifocal RGP or hydrogel lenses on both eyes. Interference and compromise with distance vision could cause the same problem as a translating bifocal. Furthermore, the RGP lens would be less comfortable initially.
3. Aspheric multifocal RGP or hydrogel lens on one eye only. A viable alternative, especially with hydrogel lenses, but a spherical correction would probably provide better near vision.

Although she adapted well, compensating glasses with a neutralizing correction for driving or a reading lens on one eye for near would have been prescribed for use with the contact lens if the patient had exhibited serious problems after a few weeks of wear. Most monovision patients feel comfortable during daylight driving, but all should be cautioned about driving at night or dusk. Relatively few seem to benefit from overcorrecting glasses whereas an equal or greater number are affected adversely by such glasses.[2] A second alternative would have been an aspheric or simultaneous vision bifocal on the left eye only. (The question of whether to charge a full fee for a one-eye fitting was anticipated by giving this patient a second lens as a spare.)

CLINICAL PEARL

The question of whether to charge a full fee for a one-eye fitting was anticipated by giving this patient a second lens as a spare.

• Case Two: Aspheric Center-Near Soft Multifocal Fitting

I. Subjective Data

A 48-year-old computer programmer presented for a bifocal correction. His habitual prescription was

OD: +2.00 − 0.50 × 085
OS: +2.25 − 0.75 × 095
Add: +2.00 D

The history revealed that he had worn hydrogel contact lenses before developing presbyopia. His present spectacles were not working well for his job environment, resulting in neck and back problems. The ocular anatomical findings showed 4 mm pupils, with the lower lid tangent to the limbus and a normal blink. He was well motivated and requested soft lenses since he felt more comfortable in that modality. The need for a correction that would allow clear vision at 24 inches directly or slightly above the midline eliminated use of any alternating segmented lens. At present there is just one soft alternating lens available; however, 13 simultaneous types, either concentric or aspheric, have been developed, and several of these might work for this patient's needs.

II. Objective Data

In this case the Unilens was selected. It is a front surface–aspheric design with maximum near power positioned centrally. The rationale for selecting a lens with a near center was based on the fact that the pupil would constrict, thus maximizing plus power under bright light conditions.

When using this lens, it is important to perform a diagnostic fitting. Remember: ± 0.25 D can affect visual acuity quite dramatically. Also "pushing plus" is advised. This lens has a usable near add of +1.75 D. During the examination, be sure to note and record the eye that will accept more plus in the distance before blur is observed. Should you then need to modify your correction and add plus power, this can be done monocularly with no loss in distance acuity of the contralateral eye. The determination of diagnostic lens prescription is as follows: from the powers of the initial lens, take half the near, add +0.25, and combine this with the distance power. The Unilens is available in base curve radii of 8.4, 8.7, 9.0, and 9.3 mm in a 14.5 mm diameter and 8.7 and 9.0 mm in a 14.0 mm diameter. My experience has been to use the 8.7 mm, 14.0 mm lens first unless the cornea is very flat or very steep. I then use several diagnostic lenses in 0.25 D steps to refine the distance prescription, ensuring that each equilibrates adequately. Since this patient had work needs at 24 inches and also had to read at 16 inches, it was important to ensure that the eye accepting more plus for distance would be overcorrected by 0.25 to

0.50 D to give the plus needed for the 16 inch reading distance. His other eye would provide acceptable vision for the 24-inch range.

III. Assessment/Plan

The following lenses were prescribed:

		BCR*	OAD	Power
OD:	Unilens	8.7 mm	14.0 mm	+3.50 D (near eye)
OS:	Unilens	8.7 mm	14.0 mm	+3.25 D (distance eye)

The patient was able to see 20/25 at distance and J4 at 16 inches. The 24-inch range was clear and solved his computer vision needs. At the follow-up visit he needed and was dispensed a +3.75 D lens for the right eye to improve his visual acuity to J2 at near, but he complained that the distance vision was now compromised. He was willing to "live with this" if there were nothing better, since it solved his problem at work.

In an effort to "optimize" this case I gave him a Simulvue 9.0 mm BCR, 14.5 mm OAD, +2.00 D lens with a 2.34 mm near center zone and a +2.50 D add for the right eye. This is also manufactured by Unilens and is a concentric multifocal with a near center in adds from +2.00 to +3.00 D. With it he now had a sharper 20/25 distance and could read J2, but he complained that the reading was not as sharp and that he initially experienced secondary images, halos, and more night reflections. He tried the Simulvue for 1 week and, surprisingly, chose to stay with it, believing that with this combination he had good binocular distance vision for driving and would be able to work at 24 inches and still have usable near vision. He realized that it was a compromise but a workable one until a more optimum lens design should become available. Maximizing the clear-vision range by utilizing multifocal soft lenses of a different type on each eye is not uncommon, since each lens has an "optical bias" at specific focal ranges.

IV. Alternative Management Plan/Summary

Obviously, many other options could have been considered, albeit with compromise. Any soft multifocal is a compromise, especially in powers that require more than +2.00 D add for near. Patients must be made aware of this and, if they are motivated, given the opportunity to try the soft multifocal. The success rate is not high, but close to half the patients who make the commitment to work with a dedicated and skilled fitter succeed. For those who fail, various rigid gas permeable (RGP) multifocals or monovision are possible options. In our practice utilizing all three modalities, the success rate for presbyopic contact lens candidates is over 80%.

---

*BCR, base curve radius; OAD, overall diameter.

• Case Three: "Occasional-Wear" Fitting Lenses

I. Subjective Data

A 55-year-old bank manager came to our office for a routine biennial examination but also was interested in being fitted with contact lenses for occasional wear when he performed as a clown for a local philanthropic organization. He was interested primarily in seeing well enough to put on his makeup and perform in public. About 10 years earlier he had been fitted with B&L PA1 aspheric multifocals for general wear but had used them only for about a year because of advancing presbyopia (that is, decreased near vision and the need for more add power).

II. Objective Data

Manifest refraction

OD: +2.00 DS (20/20) add +2.50 D (20/20)
OS: +4.25 −1.00 × 080 (20/20−) add + 2.50 D (20/20−)

Keratometry

OD: 44.50 @ 180; 45.37 @ 090 (smooth mires)
OS: 45.00 @ 180; 45.25 @ 090 (smooth mires)

Biomicroscopy

The ocular examination was unremarkable in each eye.

III. Assessment/Plan

The occasional-wear presbyopic concept with a back-surface aspheric multipack uniparameter lens has recently been introduced by Bausch & Lomb. It is designed to meet occasional and otherwise special visual needs.

To offer better binocular perception that would let him perform as well as read standard print (20/40), the Occasions multifocal lenses were selected to fit this patient over conventional monovision lenses.

 CLINICAL PEARL

As a rule, the full plus at far should always be prescribed for hyperopes.

The following throwaway diagnostic lenses were used for same-day fitting:

	Power	BCR	OAD
OD:	+2.00/less than +1.50 add*	8.7 mm	14.0 mm
OS:	+4.00/less than +1.50 add*	8.7 mm	14.0 mm

*Per manufacturer's claim.

After 10 to 15 minutes, lens centration and movement were assessed. The lenses centered well, and the patient reported them to be extremely comfortable. Initial visual acuities were 20/25 in the right eye and 20/40 in the left at both far and near, with a plano spherical overrefraction for each. To help establish a maximum occasional-wear time of 6 to 8 hours, he was encouraged to wear the new lenses to work. A supplemental half-eye spectacle prescription of +1.00 D in each eye was also dispensed for near. At 16 to 17 inches, visual acuity for both eyes was 20/20.

One week later he returned for a follow-up evaluation. His visual comfort was excellent, and he was also pleased to be able to wear his contact lenses all day (15 hours maximum), with better than expected general vision, including video display terminal functions. The +1.00 D reading prescription was extremely useful for fine print. Because of his unexpected overall satisfaction, it was recommended that he wear them on an all-day basis. Hyperopes seem to attain fairly good near acuity with these and other aspheric hydrogels, despite their limited add power.

When he returned for his final evaluation after another week, his exit visual acuities were 20/25 for the right eye, 20/30 for the left, at far and 20/40 for both eyes at near. With the spectacles he was able to read 20/20 in each eye. He was given two four-lens multipacks with a 3-month planned-replacement schedule and discharged.

IV. Alternative Management Plan/Summary

Certainly other options could have been considered, but I have found the easy-to-fit multifocal throwaway trial lenses (such as the Occasions multifocal) to be ideal for assessing the specific and occasional visual needs of many presbyopic patients. Identifying the type of use and visual expectations of a candidate at the first encounter is imperative in selecting the best multifocal contact lens.

• Case Four: Concentric Soft Bifocal for Flexible Wear

I. Subjective Data

A 44-year-old myopic salesman had been wearing hydrogel contact lenses for over 10 years. He worked with the public 85% of the time but needed to be able to write reports and enter and read information off his desktop computer. He also desired to sleep in his lenses on rare 1-night business trips. He denied having any allergies or health problems and was taking no medication other than daily multiple-vitamin supplements.

II. Objective Data

The internal examination was unremarkable. The external examination showed good lid health—a 9 mm fissure in each eye, pupil diameters of 3.0 mm by normal room lighting and 5.5 mm by dim lighting, an adequate tear meniscus, tear B.U.T. of 10+ seconds in each eye, and clear corneas.

Manifest refraction

OD: −4.00 D (20/20)
OS: −4.25 −0.50 × 010 (20/20)

Accommodative amplitude was 4.00 D, with a tentative add of 1.50 D for J2 each eye.

Keratometry

OD: 43.00 @ 180; 43.25 @ 090 (smooth mires)
OS: 43.25 @ 004; 44.00 @ 094 (smooth mires)

III. Assessment/Plan

The patient had a healthy visual system that could probably support wear of most soft bifocals. Wishing to be able to sleep in his lenses at times, he wanted very much to wear soft contact lenses. He had noted early presbyopic symptoms but was experiencing only limited visual demands in his occupation.

Initial fitting

Ciba Spectrum bifocals were selected since they offer the possibility of occasional overnight wear. The annular central near design would enable him to have natural head posture when working with his customers and also while using his computer at or about eye level.

Soft contact lens parameters

	Power	BCR	Reading zone
OD:	−3.75/+1.50 D add	8.6 mm	2.3 mm
OS:	−4.25/+1.50 D add	8.6 mm	3.0 mm

Visual acuity

OD: 20/20−(J4+)
OS: 20/25 (J4+)

Overrefraction

OD: Plano (20/20, distance) +0.75 D (J3+, near)
OS: ± 0.75 D (20/30, distance) +0.50 D (J3, near)

Biomicroscopy

The lenses centered well, and there was less than 0.5 mm movement with the blink. With a forceful blink, they moved about 1.0 mm. Using a "finger push-up" test, I found them to move smoothly and easily and to stay adequately hydrated between blinks.

At the 1-week progress evaluation he reported that distance vision with the right eye was adequate but there was a blur with the left lens. The near vision was acceptable although he had hoped for better clarity. Overrefraction found little difference from that of the dispensing visit.

At 1 month he had essentially the same complaints, and the over-refraction was similar. The following new lenses were prescribed, increasing the add power and decreasing the near zone size in his left eye.

	Power	BCR	Reading zone
OD:	−3.75 D + 2.00 D add	8.6 mm	2.3 mm
OS:	−4.25 D + 2.00 D add	8.6 mm	2.3 mm

Because he was seeing as well at near with the small reading zone in his right eye and complained only about the distance blur, a 2.3 mm zone was prescribed for the left eye as well.

Visual acuity

OD: 20/20 (J3+)
OS: 20/25+ (J3+)

Overrefraction

OD: Plano (20/20, distance) +0.50 D (J2, near)
OS: Plano (20/20, distance) +0.50 D (J2, near)

Biomicroscopy

The position and movement of these lenses were similar to those of the previous lenses. The patient stated that vision at distance was acceptable and balanced. The near-point vision was also acceptable. Minimal flare or secondary images were reported, which often occurs with concentric bifocals, especially at night as the pupil dilates.

At subsequent follow-up visits similar results were found along with good physiological tolerance of these thin medium–water content hydrogel lenses.

IV. Alternative Management Plan/Summary

If this lens proved to be inadequate, then daily use of another brand would have to be attempted. Because the patient's job required computer usage, a lens design allowing primary gaze near point was desired. Several alternate lenses could be used, including center-near aspherics like the Unilens or PS45.

CLINICAL PEARL

Spectrum is the only soft bifocal lens that can be used for overnight wear.

• Case Five: Soft Diffractive Lens Design

I. Subjective Data

A 45-year-old white woman with no prior contact lens–wearing history presented to the clinic with a desire to try contact lenses. She had received her first eyeglass prescription at her last eye examination 1 year previously. Although her spectacles were in good condition and provided good vision at distance and near, she was unhappy with her appearance and disliked wearing spectacles in general. Her position as an administrative assistant required good vision at both distance and near; she often had to greet the public. Her high motivation for contact lenses was driven primarily by the desire to maintain a positive image and by an overall dislike of glasses.

II. Objective Data

Visual acuity uncorrected

OD: 20/40 (distance)   20/100–1 (near)
OS: 20/30–2 (distance)   20/60–2 (near)

Habitual spectacle correction

OD: +2.25 DS (20/20–2, distance)   +1.00 D add (20/25–3, near)
OS: +1.75 DS (20/20+2, distance)   +1.00 D add (20/25, near)

Entrance examination

Cover test found ortho at near and far. Extraocular muscle assessment found full and unrestricted movement. The pupils were round and reactive to light, with a size estimated to be 3.5 mm in each eye. Stereo was 20 inches of arc via Randot.

Retinoscopy

OD: +3.00 DS   (20/30–1)
OS: +2.00 DS   (20/20–2)

Subjective

OD: +2.25 DS   (20/25–2)   +1.00 D add
OS: +1.75 DS   (20/20+2)   +1.00 D add

Consistent with her unremarkable visual history and entering visual acuities, no change was indicated in this patient's spectacle prescription. The objective refraction in her right eye and her measured visual acuity suggested that the preferred subjective endpoint was not the most plus.

III. Assessment/Plan

At least as important as the measured visual acuities was her acceptance of the quality of distance and near vision through overrefraction. Loose hand-held trial lenses are generally preferred for this. Subjective assessment should be made through the most plus distance endpoint combined with the lowest accepted add power. Based on these factors the following lenses were ordered:

	BCR	Power	OAD
OD:	8.7 mm	+3.00 D +1.50 D add	13.8 mm
OS:	8.7 mm	+2.25 D +1.50 D add	13.8 mm
(handling tint)		Echelon	

At the dispensing visit 1 week later, the fitting relationship and her comfort and vision were determined to be good binocularly. A hydrogen peroxide care system was dispensed, and an adaptation schedule advised. Exiting visual acuity and overrefraction with lenses were

OD: 20/25–2   Plano
OS: 20/25   –0.25 D (20/20–3, distance)

Binocular near visual acuity was 20/25, with good acceptance at near and far. The fitting relationship was judged to be similar to the diagnostic fitting. A 1-week follow-up evaluation was scheduled.

She returned 7 days later with 8 hours of lens wear that day and a maximum of 12 hours on any given day during the prior week. This wearing schedule was longer than advised at dispensing.

Visual acuity

OD: 20/25–2
OS: 20/25–1

Overrefraction

OD: Plano
OS: –0.25 D   (20/20–3)

Binocular visual acuities without overrefraction were 20/20–1 at far and 20/25 at near. She reported minimal glare, ghost images, and halos, which were explained to be normal adaptative symptoms with this lens. She was also advised that use of additional light at near as needed and positioning of the reading material at the optimum viewing distance are important.

Biomicroscopy exhibited grade 1 striae (slight corneal swelling response) in each eye with debris behind the left lens. The proper lens wearing time was discussed, in addition to the importance of proper cleaning and the use of rewetting drops to help reduce debris. If allowed to accumulate underneath the phase plate of a diffractive lens, this debris could eventually affect visual acuity. It is best managed through removal and rinsing of the lens followed by reapplication or manipulation (that is, decentering and then recentering the lens).

Since distance visual acuity was considered acceptable by the patient, no lens power changes were made. A 1-month follow-up appointment was made, and the patient was advised to hold her wearing time to no more than 12 hours per day due to the presence of striae, which were otherwise unsymptomatic.

IV. Alternative Management Plan/Summary

Obviously, other bifocal designs (rigid and hydrogel) could be considered in this case. However, the benefits of good comfort, a pupil-independent lens design, and good centration made the diffractive design preferable. This patient wore diffractive bifocal lenses, with good visual performance and no significant physiological complications, during the next 3 years before my submission of this case. Unfortunately, there were six visits during that period to replace either torn (5 visits) or lost (1 visit) lenses, which illustrates the importance of being able to provide affordable and reproducible replacement lenses to the presbyopic population in general.

• Case Six: Hydrogel Aspheric Multifocal Fitting

I. Subjective Data

A 49-year-old accountant presented to our office to be fitted with contact lenses for presbyopia in June 1993. His motivation was influenced by the visual limitations of his bifocal progressive add spectacles when using computers and various office machines. He indicated a preference for soft rather than rigid lenses.

II. Objective Data

A conventional visual analysis and ocular examination confirmed that there were no remarkable findings. His keratometric measurements and refractive findings were

Keratometry

OD: 44.25 @ 180; 45.25 @ 090 (smooth mires)
OS: 44.25 @ 180; 45.25 @ 090 (smooth mires)

Manifest refraction

OD: −1.25 −0.50 × 045   (20/20)
OS: −1.75 −0.25 × 180   (20/20)
        Add: +1.50 D

III. Assessment/Plan

He was fitted with V/X aspheric progressive-add soft lenses. Soft aspheric multifocals that are designed with the distance power in the center of the lens, and a progressive increase in plus power (the "add") 360 in each meridian from the center toward the edge are called *center distance* progressive-add aspherics.

Diagnostic lenses were used to determine whether his distance vision could be adequately corrected. Because the visual axis line is usually nasal to the geometric center of the pupil and the lens, this results in added plus power at the visual axis. It must be neutralized, and (in addition) the spherical power of refraction must be corrected. There is typically a need to add from −0.75 to −1.50 D to the distance spherical prescription. For this patient the lens power in each eye was −2.25 DS and it corrected his vision to 20/20 OU. Diagnostic lenses are essential for determining, by overrefraction, the optimum power of the ordered lenses.

CLINICAL PEARL

Because the visual axis line is usually nasal to the geometric center of the pupil and the lens, this results in added plus power at the visual axis. It must be neutralized, and (in addition) the spherical power of refraction must be corrected. There is typically a need to add from −0.75 to −1.50 D to the distance spherical prescription.

An 8.6 mm base curve radius lens was selected. However, since a hydrogel lens conforms to the corneal shape, there is no mathematical relationship between the flatter corneal meridian and the posterior apical radius (base curve) of an aspheric multifocal soft lens. The lens diameter was 14.0 mm, which is the most commonly used size.

Adaptation to the fit and correction was quite rapid and, in this case, required no reorders to obtain the desired results. Nor did the wearing of V/X soft lenses create any significant changes in the corneal curvatures or postrefraction.

IV. Alternative Management Plan/Summary

An alternative plan for this patient, considered to be an "emerging" presbyope, would have been monovision. Even with monovision, however, using the V/X soft lens instead of a standard spherical soft lens to correct near vision would have provided a better degree of distance vision and less binocular disparity. Modified "monovision" and "monoplus" are correction strategies that are ideal with aspheric soft multifocals and are being used more with advanced high-add presbyopia. The benefits of good centration, comfort, and a low to intermediate add power made the aspheric soft multifocal lens most desirable for this patient and provided intermediate as well as near add optical power.

• Case Seven: RGP Aspheric Progressive-Add Multifocals

I. Subjective Data

A 45-year-old hyperopic appliance salesman presented for fitting with contact lenses to correct presbyopia in May 1989. He had worn PMMA lenses for 20 years, and wanted contact lenses that would correct both far and near vision so he would not have to wear the heavy thick eyeglasses that his prescription required.

II. Objective Data

A conventional visual analysis and external and internal ocular examination procedures were performed. There were no remarkable findings. His prefitting keratometric measurements and subjective refraction were

Keratometry

OD: 42.25 @ 180; 43.75 @ 090 (smooth mires)
OS: 42.25 @ 180; 43.75 @ 090 (smooth mires)

Manifest refraction

OD: +8.00 DS (20/20)
OS: +8.00 −0.75 × 150 (20/40)
     Add OU: +1.50 D (J1)

III. Assessment/Plan

Because the patient was very hyperopic, his lenses had to be as thin as possible yet designed to satisfy the criteria for centration and minimal displacement on blinking. They were finally fitted 5.25 D steeper than "K" OU, which allowed them to be made thinner (less plus) and moved the center of gravity closer to the corneal plane. The front surface of each lens was made with a minus carrier lenticular design to allow the upper lid to grasp the lens better and hold it up, minimizing the typical undesired inferior positioning of high plus RGP lenses.

The posterior apical radii (base curves), powers, and sizes of the final V/X RGP aspheric corneal lenses were

	BCR	Power	OAD
OU:	47.50 D (7.10 mm)	+4.87 D	9.5 mm

Minus carrier lenticular bowl diameter, 7.5 mm

This patient achieved 20/20 distance visual acuity in each eye and near acuity of J1 (OD) and J2 (OS) with good intermediate vision as well. No lens adjustments were needed.

IV. Alternative Management Plan/Summary

Many presbyopic patients seek contact lenses that will correct their vision binocularly at all angles and distances without causing them to be aware of power changes when they switch from distance to near. They therefore seek aspheric lenses, which have the advantage over segment bifocals of being able to satisfy this need. Segment bifocal contact lenses correct near vision to below eye level, and near vision is limited to the power through the segment. RGP contact lenses that have hyperboloidal aspheric ocular surface geometries (such as the V/X) will theoretically provide up to +3.00 D for correcting near vision when the eccentricity value is 1.4 to 1.6. The near power is a function of the relationship between eccentricity and the posterior apical radius (base curve).

• Case Eight: RGP Translating Prism Ballast Lenses

I. Subjective Data

A 44-year-old man with a history of toric hydrogel and RGP wear presented for a bifocal contact lens evaluation. He had discontinued wearing his toric hydrogels because of a corneal vascularization response and his RGPs because of reduced near visual acuity. He had also attempted monovision and aspheric RGP corrections but rejected both due to visual compromises. He claimed good distance and near vision with his present progressive-addition spectacle correction; however, he desired to return to contact lens wear. His occupation demanded extensive review of documents, and therefore precise and consistent near visual performance was his major concern. Because of his repeated attempts to wear contact lenses, I considered that his motivation was high and warranted further effort.

II. Objective Data

This patient exhibited essentially normal internal and external ocular health and binocularity.

Manifest refraction

OD: −0.25 −2.00 × 161 (20/20)
OS: Plano −1.00 × 024 (20/20)
    Add: +1.50 D (20/20 OU)

Keratometry

OD: 43.25 @ 162; 45.00 @ 072 (smooth mires)
OS: 43.12 @ 021; 43.87 @ 111 (smooth mires)

By normal room lighting his pupils were 4 mm in diameter. A 12.5 mm horizontal visible iris diameter and an 11.0 mm palpebral fissure were noted with the lower lid positioned just below the inferior limbus. Note: the above anatomical dimensions are essential when considering RGP translating bifocal fitting.

III. Assessment/Plan

Hydrogel lens fitting was ruled out because of his astigmatic refractive state and past failure with monovision. In addition, past failure with simultaneous multifocal designs made a translating RGP bifocal the most viable option. I performed a diagnostic Fluoroperm ST RGP bifocal fitting utilizing a diagnostic fitting set and a base curve radius selection guide. Acceptable lens positioning translation movement, and visual acuity were obtained. Based on these results a pair of lenses were ordered with the following parameters:

	BCR	OAD/OZD*	Power/add	Prism
OD:	7.80 mm	9.4/8.0 mm	Pl/+1.50 D	1½ PD (Δ) 4.3 mm
OS:	7.82 mm	9.4/8.0 mm	+0.25/+1.50 D	1½ PD (Δ) 4.3 mm

Upon dispensing, the lenses positioned inferiorly with the segment approximately 0.4 mm below the inferior pupillary margin; 20/20 visual acuity distance and near was obtained in both eyes. Moderate lens movement with good translation on downgaze was noted, and the patient was scheduled for a follow-up visit in 1 day.

At the 1-day follow-up visit he presented having worn the lenses for approximately 2 hours and complained of fluctuating and decreased distance and near visual acuity. The lenses were riding high and positioning centrally, causing segment intersection of the visual axis. This was a lens-positioning problem and needed to be solved by lowering the lens rather than the bifocal segment height. To lower a prism translating lens, either a looser fit (flatter BCR) or an increased lens mass (increased prism ballast) can be employed. In an attempt to avoid added lens thickness with more prism, these lenses were redesigned with a flatter base curve radius by 0.50 D.

Upon dispensing, the reordered lenses exhibited acceptable fitting dynamics; however, some apical bearing and additional postblink vertical movement was noted. The patient was scheduled for a follow-up evaluation in 1 week but called the next day complaining of excessive lens movement leading to visual disruption and occasional displacement from the cornea.

A final pair of lenses was designed that returned the base curve radii to their original values and increased the prism ballast from 1.50 to 2.00 PD. Follow-up evaluations of the final lenses showed acceptable fitting dynamics, an alignment fluorescein pattern, and 20/20 visual acuity distance and near.

CLINICAL PEARL

This experience illustrates the need to obtain an alignment BCR to the corneal shape when designing Fluoroperm ST bifocal lenses. Although a flatter BCR did, in fact, lower lens positioning, it also led to excessive movement segment line interference and instability of fit. Therefore, when problem-solving lens positioning and movement related factors, it is recommended that an alignment fluorescein pattern be maintained with these types of lenses.

---

*OAD, overall diameter, OZD, optical zone diameter.

IV. Alternative Management Plan/Summary

Translating RGP bifocal contact lenses offer excellent visual performance, especially for patients with a moderate astigmatic refractive error. In general, translating designs work best for candidates who exhibit a full-time refractive correction need for both distance and near. Patient motivation is essential, because adaptation and frequent follow-up examinations are necessary. Patients who fail with hydrogel or simultaneous type RGP multifocal designs, for visual reasons, are also good candidates. However, translating designs limit near viewing to specific gazes and require more fitting expertise than simultaneous multifocal options do. In this case the Fluoroperm ST translating RGP bifocal contact lens offered improved visual performance for this patient's particular demands.

• Case Nine: Translating RGP Segmented Lens Fitting

I. Subjective Data

A 44-year-old educator at a medical center and an RGP contact lens wearer for 20 years presented with complaints of blurred distance vision, especially in dim illumination. He experienced difficulty seeing the printed titles and details on slides during lectures while wearing his present contact lenses and expressed the desire to have his vision corrected to its highest level with contact lenses.

II. Objective Data

The distance visual acuity was 20/40 in each eye but was correctable to 20/20 with the addition of −1.00 D of power over his present contact lenses. However, the additional minus power required to correct his distance vision to 20/20 blurred his near vision such that the fine print on medicine bottles became too blurred to read. Ordinary text was blurred but readable. Presbyopia was explained to him, and he was given the option of reading glasses, monovision, or bifocal contact lenses.

Ocular and anatomical measurements

Corneal diameter	11.5 mm
Lower lid to visual axis	5.25 mm
Lower lid position	0.5 mm above lower limbus
Pupil size	3.5 mm

Keratometry immediately after lens removal

OD: 39.75 @ 180; 40.25 @ 090 (smooth mires)
OS: 39.75 @ 180; 40.37 @ 090 (smooth mires)

The patient had normal healthy eyes, with normal binocular function and good stereopsis. Biomicroscopy revealed no corneal edema, stippling, striae, or neovascularization. The lids exhibited an absence of papillary hypertrophy. His present contact lenses were positioned intrapalpebral, and the fluorescein pattern showed alignment in the optical zone with peripheral clearance in all meridians.

His present CAB contact lenses measured

	BCR	Power	OAD/OZD	CT
OD:	8.55 mm	−2.25 D	8.8/7.8 mm	0.20 mm
OS:	8.55 mm	−1.75 D	8.8/7.8 mm	0.20 mm

III. Assessment/Plan

The existing lens/cornea fitting relationship was good, and it was decided that the new translating bifocals should be similar to his present lenses. The same base curve radii were selected, making the appropriate power modifications and allowing for a bifocal power of +1.50 D in the segment.

Diagnostic lens fitting

The flattest base curve–radius lens in the standard available diagnostic fitting set was selected and measured 8.23 mm BCR, −2.00/+2.00 D add, 2 Δ, 9.4 × 9.0 mm OAD, and 4.2 mm seg height. This lens was placed on the right eye and positioned well, with the truncation supported by the lower lid. It translated well on downgaze and showed the effect of nasal up torque, rotating slightly counterclockwise with the blink. The fluorescein pattern exhibited central pooling, confirming the fact that this lens was 1.25 D steeper than K. An overrefraction of −2.75 D was required to obtain 20/20 vision. The 4.2 mm segment height was judged to be high; 4.0 mm would be preferable.

This same diagnostic lens was placed on the left eye, and similar observations were made. The lens positioned well on the lower lid, was supported by the lower lid, and translated smoothly on downgaze. Nasal torque caused it to rotate slightly clockwise with the blink. The fluorescein pattern showed central pooling, the 4.2 mm segment was too high, and an overrefraction of −2.25 D was required to obtain 20/20 vision.

Measurements were made to determine the bifocal height by observing that the normal lower lid position was 0.5 mm above the limbus and the distance from the lower lid margin to the visual axis was 5.25 mm. The bifocal was designed to be 1.25 mm below the visual axis, resulting in a 4 mm segment height. The vertical height of the lens was determined by measuring the distance from where the lower lid intersected the cornea (0.5 mm above lower limbus) to the superior limbus and allowing at least 2 mm (from the apex of the lens to the superior limbus) for a smooth upward translation of the lens on downgaze. A standard 0.4 mm truncation was used for lid support, and the lens diameter was specified as 9.4 × 9.0 mm. Prism ballast was ordered 2 pd standard, with the axis 15° nasal to the 90° meridian in each eye to counteract the nasal torque induced by blinking.

Contact lens specifications

Tangent Streak bifocals were ordered with the following specifications:

	BCR	Power	OAD	Seg height
OD:	8.55 mm	−3.25 D +1.50 D Add × 105	9.4 × 9.0 mm	4.0 mm
OS:	8.55 mm	−2.75 D +1.50 D Add × 075	9.4 × 9.0 mm	4.0 mm

The initial visual results were excellent. The patient could read the distance 20/20 line with each eye, and the fine print on the back of a medicine bottle was clear. The lenses positioned and performed well, with the following exceptions: at times they were lifted by the upper lid with the blink, causing the distance vision to blur momentarily as the visual axis passed through the add segment; in addition, occasionally they would not translate upward but would slide under the lower lid on downgaze so the visual axis continued to pass through the distance segment and the near vision was blurred.

The diagnosis was: Excessive lens lifting and inconsistant translation. Modifications were made to correct these problems.

1. The lid-caused lens lift was addressed by adding a front surface bevel to only the superior and lateral areas of the lens periphery (from 9 through 12 to 3 o'clock) using a 90° tool and rocking the lens as the tool was applied to it to blend the bevel smoothly onto its front surface curve. This had the effect of reducing peripheral mass and the edges of the segment ledge as well as changing the vector forces of the lid on the superior area of the lens so the lens would no longer be lifted by the normal opening of the blink. (This "lifting" effect is most frequently observed with thick or thick-edged lenses as the upper lid engages the lens and displaces it upward.)

2. The failure of this lens to properly translate to the near segment on downgaze was addressed by modifying the truncation using a flat disc tool and holding the lens tilted 15° toward the ocular surface so it would not slide beneath the lower lid.

Note: When the truncation is modified, care must be taken to reapply the peripheral curve radius to the truncated area to maintain comfort and allow the lens to quickly resume its position of rest on the lower lid.

This fitting was accomplished in March 1986. The patient has returned for annual visits, at which time the lenses have been cleaned and polished. His last visit was January 1994, and he remarkably continues to wear the original lenses, maintaining 20/20 visual acuity at distance and near. The RGP translating neonocentric design of the taugent streak is still current and unique to this day, and is frequently prescribed.

IV. Alternative Management Plan/Summary

The development of higher–oxygen transmission rigid gas-permeable (RGP) polymers has allowed greater freedom of optical design without compromising corneal physiology in the custom fitting of prism-ballasted, translating, bifocal contact lenses. The Tangent Streak bifocal was selected for this patient because it provided an opportunity to duplicate the vision that could be obtained with traditional bifocal spectacle lenses. The Tangent Streak can also be designed over a wide range of refractive errors and corneal curvatures although it requires learned skills in fitting measuring and modifying the RGP material.

• Case Ten: RGP Translating Bifocal Contact Lens

I. Subjective Data

A healthy 66-year-old housewife came to our office desiring bifocal contact lenses. She had been fitted with polymethyl methacrylate (PMMA) monovision lenses 16 years earlier. The doctor who had fitted her originally had since retired and the doctor who assumed his practice did not desire to fit contact lenses. She was wearing her lenses for approximately 12 hours daily but felt that the vision was not as good as she would like; she was visually insecure at night, and her vision would become increasingly difficult the longer she wore her lenses. She reported that after wearing the lenses her vision with glasses was very poor.

II. Objective Data

Unaided visual acuity

OD: 20/200
OS: 20/200
OU: 20/200

Visual acuity with current contact lenses

OD: 20/30
OS: 20/60

Overrefraction

OD: +1.25 –0.50 × 090 (20/20)
OS: –0.75 –0.50 × 095 (20/20)

Current contact lens parameters

	BCR	OAD	Power
OD:	7.70 mm	9.0 mm	+3.00 D
OS:	7.70 mm	9.0 mm	+5.50 D

Manifest refraction

OD: +4.25 –1.50 × 090 (20/20) add: +2.50 D
OS: +4.25 –1.00 × 095 (20/20) add: +2.50 D

Keratometry

OD: 42.37 @ 090; 44.50 @ 180 (slight mire distortion)
OS: 42.75 @ 090; 44.50 @ 180 (slight mire distortion)

External appearance

All structures were normal, with palpebral fissures measuring 10 mm
vertically and a horizontal corneal diameter of 12 mm. The lower lid
was 0.5 mm above the lower limbus. The pupil size was 3.5 mm by
room illumination. A complete blink was present.

Biomicroscopy

Both eyes manifested +1 central corneal clouding and early lenticular
changes.

Diagnosis and treatment

1. Corneal edema and curvature deformation due to long-term
   PMMA contact lens wear
2. Presbyopia undercorrected with present contact lenses for monovision and residual (lenticular) astigmatism correction

III. Assessment/Plan

After a discussion of the causes of some of her problems, we mutually
agreed to refit her with rigid gas-permeable (RGP) contact lenses. I
explained to her the need for wearing prism-ballast lenses in a bifocal
design to reduce the residual astigmatism and provide near vision,
and we eventually decided to fit her with Tangent Streak RGP
bifocals.

Diagnostic fitting

	BCR	OAD/OZD	Power/add	Seg height
OU:	7.70 mm	9.6(H),9.4(V)/8.2 mm	+5.00/+1.75 D	4.5 mm

Biomicroscopy

The fluorescein pattern exhibited an alignment fit with the expected
against-the-rule pattern. The bifocal segment was approximately 0.4
mm too high in straight-ahead gaze, and on downgaze there was
adherence at the superior limbus that prevented full translation.
Therefore, when ordering the initial lenses, the overall diameter and
segment height were reduced. The overrefraction at distance was

OD: –0.75 DS (20/20)
OS: –0.50 DS (20/20)

The following Tangent Streak Fluorex 700 lenses were ordered:

	BCR/SCR/PCR(W)*	OAD/OZD	Power
OD:	7.65/8.75/11.25 (0.2 mm)	9.2(H),9.0(V)/8.0 mm	+4.00 D
OS:	7.65/8.75/11.00 (0.2 mm)	9.2(H),9.0(H)/8.0 mm	+4.25 D
	Add: +2.00 D Prism: 2.25 Δ Seg height: 4.1 mm		

At the dispensing visit her visual acuity and comfort were initially good.

Visual acuity (distance and near)

OD: 20/25/ J2
OS: 20/25/ J2

Overrefraction

OD: Plano
OS: −0.25 D

Corneal alignment was present with an against-the-rule pattern at fluorescein evaluation. The lenses were positioned inferiorly, with truncation riding on the lower lid margin.

At the 2-week visit her right eye felt good, but she said the left lens was still a little irritating. Her vision was good, and the wearing time was up to 12 hours.

Visual acuity (distance/near)

OD: 20/20/ J1
OS: 20/20/ J1

Overrefraction

OD: Plano
OS: −0.25 D

Biomicroscopy

Light and diffuse 3 and 9 o'clock staining OU was observed; otherwise the eyes were clear.

Modifications

The secondary curve radius was flattened to 8.85 mm; a heavy blend was applied as well.

At the 5-week visit no problems had occurred with comfort or vision. She had some dryness, and her wearing time was still 12 hours/day. Visual acuity and biomicroscopy were unchanged from the previous visit.

She was instructed to use rewetting drops if dryness became a problem. At this point I believed she would be successful, and she was

---

*BCR, base curve radius; SCR, secondary curve radius; PCR, peripheral curve radius.

released for 6 months. It has now been 3 years that she has worn the lenses, and she has not had any significant problems.

IV. Alternative Management Plan/Summary

Several other options were available to this patient, but none would have provided as good vision and oxygen transmissibility as the lenses that were selected. These included
1. Soft astigmatic lenses for distance with spectacles for near
2. Prism-ballast RGPs for distance with spectacles for near
3. Astigmatic soft monovision lenses
4. RGP prism-ballast monovision lenses
5. Aspheric RGP bifocal lenses

This was a straightforward RGP translating bifocal fitting. Not all fittings are this routine; most require some modification in lens design or peripheral curves during the fitting period. However, by performing all the steps required in a meticulous diagnostic fitting, the practitioner can reduce the number of remakes and overall cost. Some "pearls" for fitting Tangent Streak bifocals are given in the box.

TANGENT STREAK FITTING "PEARLS"

- *Previous rigid lens wearers adapt well to these bifocal lenses.*
- *Be sure that the patient has tight lower lids positioned at or slightly above the lower limbus.*
- *Patients with high ametropia usually adapt better than those with low ametropia.*
- *Patients with small pupil diameters are less problematical than those with larger pupils.*
- *Always keep in mind the patient's vision needs—people who spend long hours on a computer will not be best served by a translating bifocal.*
- *Generally patients who have a with-the-rule astigmatism perform better than those who are against-the-rule.*
- *When prescribing an add, take the power you would prescribe for spectacles and reduce it 0.25 or 0.50 D to obtain the add for these lenses.*

• Case Eleven: Lifestyle Hi-Rider

I. Subjective Data

A 44-year-old homemaker who said she "reads constantly" had successfully worn spherical Polycon II RGP lenses for 11 years. She presented in the office with complaints of increased myopic shift, especially her left eye, along with presbyopic changes. She was taking clonidine for essential hypertension and also reported that she had seasonal allergies but these did not disrupt her ability to wear RGP lenses throughout the year. She was wearing the lenses all her waking hours and rarely used her glasses for backup. She had successfully worn PMMA lenses since 1965 until she was refitted into RGP lenses in 1982. There had been no previous corneal distortion or significant ocular health changes with her Polycon II lenses.

II. Objective Data

Visual acuity with Polycon II lenses

OD: 20/20
OS: 20/30

Overrefraction

OD: −0.25 DS (20/20)
OS: −1.00 DS (20/20)

Current contact lens parameters

	BCR	Power	OAD/OZD	Tint
OD:	7.65 mm	−2.00 D	9.0/7.6 mm	Blue no. 1
OS:	7.65 mm	−1.75 D	9.0/7.6 mm	Blue no. 1

Biomicroscopy

The biomicroscopy examination revealed lids, lashes, conjunctiva, and cornea to be free of ocular pathology.

Manifest refraction (½ hour after lens removal)

OD: −3.00 −0.50 × 180 (20/20)
OS: −3.00 −0.50 × 180 (20/20)
Add +1.25 D OU

Automated keratometry

OD: 44.25 @ 170; 45.37 @ 80 degrees (smooth mires)
OS: 44.62 @ 174; 45.00 @ 84 degrees (smooth mires)

III. Assessment/Plan

She was successfully fitted with Lifestyle Hi-Riders in the SGP II material.

	BCR (equiv)	Power	OAD	CT	Tint
OD:	EQ* 7.70 mm	−3.00 D	9.00 mm	0.16 mm	Blue no. 1
OS:	EQ 7.60 mm	−3.25 D	9.00 mm	0.16 mm	Blue no. 1

Three factors are important in fitting this lens: keratometry, fluorescein biomicroscopy assessment, and lacrimal evaluation (tear B.U.T.). She demonstrated normal ocular corneal measurements, including an 11.5 mm corneal diameter with a 10.0 mm palpebral

---

*EQ stands for *equalized base curve*, a new concept in contact lens fitting. (Refer to Hansen DW: *Contact Lens Spectrum*, October 1993.)

fissure. Her pupil size under mesopic conditions was 4.0 mm, and under scotopic conditions 5.0 mm, in each eye.

She was an early presbyope with ocular physical characteristics within the normal range. Presbyopic patients often have a reduced tear film, which usually does not preclude fitting the lens. Her diagnosis of early presbyopia, ocular measurements that fell within the normally expected range, and previously demonstrated ability to wear RGP lenses were the three criteria that convinced me she would be a suitable candidate for Lifestyle Hi-Riders. These lenses are made with an aspheric back surface that allows the patient to see comfortably at distance, near, and intermediate ranges.

The unique aspherical back surface design allows the Lifestyle Hi-Riders to perform more like alternating vision lenses, without the need for low positioning. The lid-attachment characteristics give these lenses the "Hi-Rider" name and greatly improve their translation from distance to intermediate to near. The SGP II rigid gas-permeable material provides a physiologically safe lens to protect the eye and adnexa. Hi-Riders come in 9.0 and 9.5 mm sizes. For this patient we decided on a 9.0 mm design, similar to her previous 9.0 mm Polycons. Her lid characteristics (that is, a smaller than average eye and normal eyelid configuration) helped in the selection process.

Selecting the appropriate base curve radius is a factor in achieving success. It is important to follow the normal rules for proper vertical lens movement on the cornea whether it is flat or steep. For patients with a corneal toricity less than 1.5 D, the lens should be fitted 0.1 mm flatter than "K." This will allow the lens to decenter superiorly and aid the lid attachment in higher myopic prescriptions (Plate 11).

The lens is fitted by means of a system called equalized base curve (EQ). Keratometry should be used to determine the base curve radius

---

Preselection Evaluation Tests

Case history
    Assess motivation
Occupational or avocational demands
    Determine computer usage
Ocular characteristics
    Fissure size
    Pupil assessment (mesopic and scotopic)
    Blink rate/quality
    Lacrimal assessment (tear B.U.T. and meniscus)
    Eyelid measurements (tonicity and position)
    Pupil-to-lid measurement
    Keratometric readings

necessary to fit the lens approximately 0.50 D flatter than "K." This number is converted to the proper EQ value using the conversion chart provided by Permeable Technologies. (The philosophy of fitting a lens flatter than normal aspheric designs is unique; other aspheric designs fit from 1.50 to 4.00 D *steeper* than "K.")

After a diagnostic lens is selected, a spherocylinder overrefraction should be performed and placed in a trial frame to determine the overall translation of the vision from far to near. If excessive translation causes problems with distance and near visual acuity, a different base curve radius should be selected to maximize visual acuity. To raise the lens superiorly, a larger diameter with a flatter base curve is needed. Conversely, if the lens needs to move inferiorly in a more central location, the base curve radius should be steepened and the diameter decreased to 9.0 mm.

This patient returned for a follow-up examination seeing 20/20+ and J1 in each eye at near. She enjoyed the comfort, and the translation from far to near was acceptable for her daily activities.

IV. Alternative Management Plan/Summary

This patient's early presbyopia allowed for a number of options that could satisfy her needs. (The box offers criteria that are beneficial in determining RGP bifocal selection based on a patient's occupational and leisure activities.) Since she did not work with computers, almost any bifocal style would be appropriate. It is commonplace to fit aspheric lenses or simultaneous-vision lenses on patients with an intermediate demand. Computer users have this type of demand, and it is appropriate to fit them with aspheric or simultaneous designs to enhance their intermediate zone.

CLINICAL PEARL

It is commonplace to fit aspheric lenses or simultaneous-vision lenses on patients with an intermediate demand. Computer users have this type of demand, and it is appropriate to fit them with aspheric or simultaneous designs to enhance their intermediate zone.

Other options for this patient included monovision contact lenses and spectacles worn over contact lenses for near activities. Because of the relative ease of fitting aspheric designs, it was decided to perform a diagnostic lens examination with these lenses. Bifocal contact lenses enhanced her binocularity, which was especially helpful for her favorite pastime (reading).

• Case Twelve: Multisite Aspheric Bifocal Design

I. Subjective Data

A 43-year-old insurance payroll analyst presented in the office complaining of near blurriness, especially when using the computer for an extended time. She had been wearing spherical hydrogel W-J Aquaflex lenses to correct her moderately high myopic condition.

	BCR	Power	OAD
OD:	Vault III 8.20 mm	−6.75 D	13.2 mm
OS:	Vault III 8.20 mm	−6.50 D	13.2 mm

She had been diagnosed with lupus erythematosus but was in a remissive state at this time. She complained of dimness of vision, dry eyes, and glare with light at night, accompanied by near visual blurriness. She was taking six aspirin per day, along with calcium and vitamins, to control the lupus. She had no known allergies to environmental conditions, chemicals, foods, or drugs. The external examination revealed her pupils to be equal, round, and responsive to light and accommodation.

II. Objective Data

She presented for the visual examination with an overrefraction of −0.50 D over both her hydrogel lenses, resulting in a visual acuity of 20/20 in each eye. A +1.00 D add was necessary to correct her presbyopia. Her lids, lashes, conjunctiva, and corneas revealed no ocular pathology. A baseline refraction was performed after removal of her hydrogel lenses.

Manifest refraction

OD: −9.25 −0.25 × 180 (20/20)
OS: −9.25 −0.75 × 130 (20/20)

She demonstrated a 4.0 mm pupil diameter under mesopic conditions, and a 5.0 mm pupil under scotopic conditions, in both eyes. The corneal diameter was 12.0 mm with a 10.0 mm palpebral fissure.

III. Assessment/Plan

This woman was an early presbyope who had been given increased near-point tasks because of her employment and who used a computer approximately 100% of the day. The intermediate zone was very important for her daily needs. Some practitioners would express concern over changing a patient from daily-wear hydrogel lenses to a rigid gas-permeable material; however, this was not a major concern. Once the options were explained, she was willing to proceed with a diagnostic appointment for RGP bifocal lenses to evaluate the potential for change.

Lupus erythematosus is a collagen vascular disease, an inflammatory connective tissue disorder of unknown etiology, occurring predominantly in young women. Fibrinoid necrosis and bodies of altered nuclear material may be found in the tissues of any organ. Her systemic condition was an integral part of our lens selection process as well as my design of her contact lenses. Because it was in remission, I deemed her an appropriate candidate for RGP aspheric simultaneous-vision lenses to improve her acuity, especially in the midrange, and also to provide overall comfort with the non–prism ballast design.

The Multisite lens requires good centration for success and is usually fitted 2.75 to 4.00 D steeper than "K" depending on the amount of corneal astigmatism. The distance segment of the lens is 3 mm on the geometrical center, the average diameter 9.3 mm, and the maximum effective addition +2.25 D. It is now possible, through computerized lathes specialized, to generate additional plus on the front surface of the lens.

Keratometry

OD: 44.75 @ 173; 45.37 @ 083
OS: 45.12 @ 158; 45.87 @ 068

Because of her low corneal toricity, a lens 3.00 D steeper than "K" was selected as the diagnostic lens. The spherocylinder refraction and lens positioning assessment via biomicroscopy showed good centering with a slight lag in each eye. The fluorescein pattern of this particular design provided a bulls-eye appearance due to the steepness of the lens eccentricity (Plate 12).

This extra pooling in the central zone typically does not produce a physiologically poor fit but allows the practitioner to evaluate the distance segment over the pupil. It is very important to have a well-centered lens. If the overrefraction results in a need for –0.75 D or more power, the practitioner should suspect a poorly positioned lens. In addition, the presence of greater than 0.75 D residual astigmatism usually contraindicates this lens for a patient.

She was fitted with the following lens design:

	BCR	Power	OAD/OZD	SCR	PCR(W)	CT
OD:	7.06 mm	–11.00 D	9.5/8.3 mm	9.00 mm	11.50 (0.4 mm)	0.17 mm
OS:	7.03 mm	–11.00 D	9.5/8.3 mm	9.00 mm	11.50 (0.4 mm)	0.17 mm
OU:	Paraperm 02 material, Blue no. 1					

These lenses are manufactured with an aspheric eccentricity value (to create a +1.50 D add) by Salvatori Ophthalmics. The patient was examined 10 days after the dispensing and reported no symptoms. She was seeing 20/20+ in each eye and J1 for near individually. Wearing the lenses 14 to 16 hours per day, she reported improved vision at all ranges and said they were as "comfortable now as her

---

Troubleshooting the Multisite

Poor distance acuity
   Check horizontal and vertical alignment; may require steeper or flatter base curve to achieve centering.
   Check for poor blinking.
   Reduce lens diameter if too much lid involvement.
   Add additional power for distance, check near point.
Poor near vision
   Check for lower lid capture on downward gaze; size reduction should help.
   Design with more add.
   Increase add power to existing lens.
Poor distance and near
   Check overrefraction and add of existing lens.
   Change residual cylinder design.
   Check for soiled or filmy lens.

---

former soft lenses." The adaptation period was short, probably because of the improved vision. (See box.)

IV. Alternative Management Plan/Summary

Patients using computers for lengthy periods, at work or at home, are excellent candidates for simultaneous-vision lenses. Translating bifocals are usually not appropriate because of the void at intermediate ranges. Her options included monovision contact lenses and reading spectacles made for the computer distance and worn over hydrogel lenses. Because of the intensity of her work, binocularity was extremely important and she adapted exceptionally well to the conversion.

Bifocal contact lens designs have expanded greatly over the years, and materials and manufacturing technology now exist to accompany their consistently reliable parameters. Accurate preselection and education of patients will enhance wider public and professional acceptance of multifocal contact lenses.

Bibliography

1. London R: Monovision correction for diplopia, *J Am Optom Assoc* 58:568-570, 1987.
2. Pence NA: Monovision and driving. Presented at the North American Research Symposium, San Diego, August 1993.

8

Management of Diseased and Postsurgical Corneas

Larry J. Davis

Optical rehabilitation for the patient with corneal disease can be one of the most rewarding of patient encounters. Often the individual has experienced numerous failed attempts to achieve a clear and comfortable alternative elsewhere. Most have a strong motivation for optimal vision performance. Thus their desire to proceed with the prescribed therapy is higher than for patients who do not stand to obtain such benefits. Therefore, one of the most important predictors of success with contact lens wear, *patient motivation,* is usually quite high. When success is apparent, the practitioner is rewarded through a feeling of "job well done," along with the trust and loyalty of patients and their families into the future.

The *art* and *science* of prescribing spectacles and contact lenses for the irregular cornea require an extra level of expertise beyond that necessary for more routine patient encounters. Fortunately, the numerous lens designs currently available allow for a high rate of success. Appropriate contact lens parameters are available for virtually all clinical presentations. Therefore an absence of visual clarity is rarely the primary factor for patient dissatisfaction. More often factors that limit successful contact lens correction in patients with diseased corneas are stability of lens fit, lens awareness, or lens care and insertion/removal difficulties. The following cases include strategies for management of such challenging patients. With regard to various diseases that affect the cornea, diagnostic criteria have been omitted because of space limitations. Strategies for management are emphasized.

• Case One: Incipient Keratoconus

I. Subjective Data

A 32-year-old woman with a 12-year history of soft contact lens wear presented with the complaint of blurred distance vision in her left eye for the past few months that seemed to be worsening. She had not had any prior trauma or surgery and was taking no medications.

II. Objective Data

Visual acuity

		BCR*	Power
OD:	Hydron Mini	8.50 mm	−2.50 D (20/25)
OS:	Hydron Mini	8.50 mm	−2.50 D (20/50)

Overrefraction

OD: −0.25 D (20/20)
OS: −0.25 D (20/30)

Current spectacle prescription

OD: −2.25 DS
OS: −2.75 DS

Manifest refraction

OD: −2.75 −0.50 × 080 (20/20)
OS: −3.25 −1.25 × 135 (20/40, indistinct endpoint)

Cycloplegic refraction

OD: −1.75 −0.50 × 175 (20/20)
OS: −1.25 −1.25 × 135 (20/40)

Keratometry

OD: 44.00 @ 180; 44.50 @ 090 (smooth mires)
OS: 43.50 @ 150; 45.25 @ 060 (slight distortion)

Biomicroscopy

The contact lenses centered well, with 2 to 3 mm of movement. The lids, lashes, and conjunctivae were clear, and the corneas showed no striae or Fleischer's rings. Fingerprint dystrophy changes were observed near the inferior limbus of the left eye. She was instructed to discontinue contact lens wear for 10 days and to return for follow-up.

---

*BCR, base curve radius.

At the follow-up visit 10 days later I found:

Manifest refraction

OD: −2.00 −0.50 × 015 (20/20)
OS: −2.50 −0.75 × 145 (20/20)

Keratometry

OD: 43.63 @ 015; 44.50 @ 105 (smooth mires)
OS: 43.87 @ 175; 45.50 @ 085 (slight distortion)

She was refitted with a spherical soft contact lens (Durasoft 3) for the right eye and a soft toric lens (D2 Optifit) for the left. Seven months later she had no complaints.

Manifest refraction

OD: −2.75 −0.50 × 015 (20/20)
OS: −3.25 −1.25 × 160 (20/20)

Three months after that she complained of blur in the left eye for the preceding 2 weeks.

Visual acuity with contact lenses

OD: 20/20
OS: 20/50

Manifest refraction

OD: −2.25 −0.50 × 010 (20/20)
OS: −3.75 −1.50 × 170 (20/25)

Keratometry

OD: 44.00 @ 180; 45.00 @ 090 (smooth mires)
OS: 44.25 @ 165; 47.00 @ 075 (slightly distorted mires)

EyeSys videokeratography showed marked steepening beneath the visual axis in the left eye, suggestive of early keratoconus (Plate 13).

Biomicroscopy

A partial Fleischer's ring was observed in the left eye. This eye was then refitted with a toric lens having a higher spherical and cylindrical power consistent with the above refraction.

She returned as requested for routine follow-up 9 months later (19 months after the initial examination) complaining that her visual acuity was not as sharp.

Visual acuity with contact lenses

OD: 20/20
OS: 20/30

Manifest refraction

OD: −3.00 (20/20)
OS: −4.25 (20/20)

Keratometry

OD: 43.25 DS (smooth mires)
OS: 44.00 @ 165; 45.37 @ 075 (slightly distorted mires)

She was refitted with spherical soft contact lenses, which she continued to wear for the next year. EyeSys videokeratography showed values similar to the baseline visit.

III. Assessment/Plan

Contact lens wear may be associated with changes in corneal and refractive astigmatism. Astute clinicians will often suspect the presence of contact lens–induced corneal warpage in wearers who have a reduced best corrected spectacle visual acuity along with an indistinct endpoint refraction. Other causes of irregular corneal astigmatism, including surface disease (such as dry eye) and corneal ectatic disease (such as keratoconus or pellucid marginal degeneration), also need to be considered. After removal of the contact lenses for 10 days the endpoint refraction was more distinct and visual acuity in the affected eye returned to 20/20. Therefore, in the absence of other definitive clinical signs suggesting keratoconus, it was presumed that the etiology of her symptoms was contact lens overwear. However, when her symptoms returned 10 months later, she had developed a subtle Fleischer's ring, which is a definitive clinical sign of keratoconus. Isolated steepening of the inferior half of the cornea as demonstrated by computer-assisted videokeratography further supported this diagnosis.

IV. Alternative Management Plan/Summary

This case was unusual in that, despite persistence of slight distortion of the keratometer mires 19 months after her initial presentation, a reduction of refractive astigmatism allowed for a more simple spherical contact lens. Furthermore, it demonstrated that RGP contact lenses are not necessary for all keratoconus patients. Often the novice contact lens practitioner is accustomed to considering a rigid lens alternative whenever keratoconus is suspected. Although one could not be faulted for prescribing a rigid lens in such a case, continuation of soft lens wear is probably easier for the patient already adapted to soft contact lenses. Patients with early keratoconus may see very well with soft toric lenses. When the visual acuity through soft lenses is compromised (as demonstrated by best spectacle visual acuity) RGP contact lenses should be considered.

• Case Two: Advanced Keratoconus

I. Subjective Data

A 34-year-old man with a 16-year history of keratoconus was referred for contact lens refitting. He complained of marked lens awareness daily after 3 to 4 hours of contact lens wear that had begun approximately 4 months earlier. His last eye examination had been 5 years ago, when his present lenses were fitted. He had no complaints regarding visual acuity or the stability of lens fit.

II. Objective Data

Visual acuity with contact lenses

OD: 20/25
OS: 20/30

Overrefraction

OD: −0.25 D (no improvement)
OS: −0.50 D (20/20)

Contact lens parameters

	BCR	OAD/OZD*	Power
OD:	7.5 mm	9.6/8.2 mm	−3.00 D
OS:	7.5 mm	9.6/8.2 mm	−2.50 D

The surfaces were clear, with few superficial scratches and deposits.

Biomicroscopy

The contact lenses were positioned under the upper lid (Korb fit) with 2 to 3 mm of blink-induced movement. Fluorescein revealed a marked central touch with excessive edge lift (Plate 14). The lids and lashes showed blepharitis, with inspissated Meibomian glands in each eye. The conjunctivae were clear, but both corneas had Fleischer's rings and striae. Punctate staining was observed in the central corneas, with central anterior stromal scarring in the right eye (Plate 15). The anterior chambers and crystalline lenses were clear.

Keratometry

OD: 52.37 @ 165; 56.00 @ 075 (smooth mires)
OS: 50.00 @ 010; 55.50 @ 100 (smooth mires)

Manifest refraction

OD: −11.00 −2.50 × 150 (20/70)
OS: −9.75 −4.00 × 15 (20/60)

---

*Overall diameter/optical zone diameter.

III. Assessment/Plan

This patient was wearing RGP contact lenses that had been fitted 5 years previously. Disease progression during that period had promoted increased corneal ectasia with resultant steepening of the corneal curvatures. Thus a markedly flat base curve/cornea fitting relationship was observed. The central touch and excessive edge lift were associated with lens awareness due to mechanical rubbing of the corneal epithelium.

Visual acuity is usually minimally affected in such cases. Management is aimed at providing a more uniform distribution of contact lens/corneal touch. Refitting is performed by utilizing rigid diagnostic contact lenses designed for these unique curvatures. As a rule such lenses have steeper posterior apical radii, with smaller overall and optical zone diameters and higher axial edge lift peripheral curves (Table 8-1).

For refitting, the initial base curve radius was chosen as the flattest keratometric value. Careful observation of the tear dye pattern was utilized for adjustment of the posterior apical radius (PAR), optical zone diameter, and peripheral curve design (Plate 16). The final lens parameters were:

	PAR	OAD/OZD	Power
OD:	6.49 mm	8.5/6.5 mm	−10.00 D
OS:	6.62 mm	8.5/6.5 mm	−9.00 D

TABLE 8-1
Sample Keratoconus Fitting Set*

PAR (mm)	Power (D)	OAD/OZD (mm)	SCR(W) (mm)	PCR(W) (mm)
8.03(42.00)	3.00	9.0/7.0	9.0(0.7)	12.0(0.3)
7.85(43.00)	3.00	9.0/7.0	9.0(0.7)	12.0(0.3)
7.67(44.00)	3.00	9.0/7.0	9.0(0.7)	12.0(0.3)
7.50(45.00)	3.00	9.0/7.0	9.0(0.7)	12.0(0.3)
7.34(46.00)	3.00	9.0/7.0	9.0(0.7)	12.0(0.3)
7.18(47.00)	3.00	9.0/7.0	9.0(0.7)	12.0(0.3)
7.03(48.00)	3.00	9.0/7.0	9.0(0.7)	12.0(0.3)
6.89(49.00)	6.00	8.5/6.5	9.0(0.7)	12.0(0.3)
6.75(50.00)	6.00	8.5/6.5	9.00(0.7)	12.0(0.3)
6.62(51.00)	6.00	8.5/6.5	9.0(0.7)	12.0(0.3)
6.49(52.00)	6.00	8.5/6.5	9.0(0.7)	12.0(0.3)
6.37(53.00)	6.00	8.5/6.5	9.0(0.7)	12.0(0.3)
6.25(54.00)	12.00	8.5/6.0	9.0(0.8)	12.0(0.45)
6.14(55.00)	12.00	8.5/6.0	9.0(0.8)	12.0(0.45)
6.03(56.00)	12.00	8.5/6.0	9.0(0.8)	12.0(0.45)
5.92(57.00)	12.00	8.0/6.0	9.0(0.7)	12.0(0.3)
5.82(58.00)	16.00	8.0/6.0	9.0(0.7)	12.0(0.3)
5.72(59.00)	16.00	8.0/6.0	9.0(0.7)	12.0(0.3)
5.62(60.00)	16.00	8.0/6.0	9.0(0.7)	12.0(0.3)

*The material should be PMMA or a low-Dk rigid gas-permeable plastic.

The peripheral curves in each eye were

PCR(W)* = 13.0 (0.3 mm)
ICR(W) = 9.0 (0.7 mm)

IV. Alternative Management Plan/Summary

Keratoconus may present with a wide variety of corneal shapes and irregularities as well as numerous degrees, positions, and sizes of ectatic-induced steepening representing a wide spectrum of disease. Classification systems based on the size of ectasia and the topographic shape have been introduced. Although these often prove beneficial, most keratoconus patients have corneas that do not fit particularly well with such general classification criteria. Thus a "cookbook" approach to fitting corneas with advanced keratoconus is not possible. Furthermore, experienced fitters in this area do not agree on the optimal lens design and/or fitting relationship for keratoconus. However, a few general strategies will assist the fitter with improving contact lens fit (Fig. 8-1).

1. Begin to visualize two corneal fitting zones. In moderate to advanced keratoconus the *central* 5 to 7 mm, which includes the visual axis, has a shape quite different from that of the *peripheral* zones. Furthermore, the transition between ectatic corneal substance and substance that is less affected by disease often shows a dramatic change from steep to flat.

2. Steeper central corneal curvatures require shorter posterior apical radii with smaller overall and optical zone diameters. Optical zone diameters larger than 7 mm and overall diameters larger than 9.0 mm are the exception once posterior apical radii of 7 mm or less are required to fit the central cornea. When radii of 6.5 mm and less are required, optical zone diameters of 6.0 mm should be considered. Optical zones smaller than 6.0 mm often induce significant glare and, with few exceptions, should be avoided.

CLINICAL PEARL

Steeper central corneal curvatures require shorter posterior apical radii with smaller overall and optical zone diameters.

3. In general, constant peripheral curve radii and widths, regardless of the posterior apical radius, provide an excellent *initial design*. A

---

*PCR(W), peripheral curve radius (with width); ICR(W), intermediate curve radius (with width).

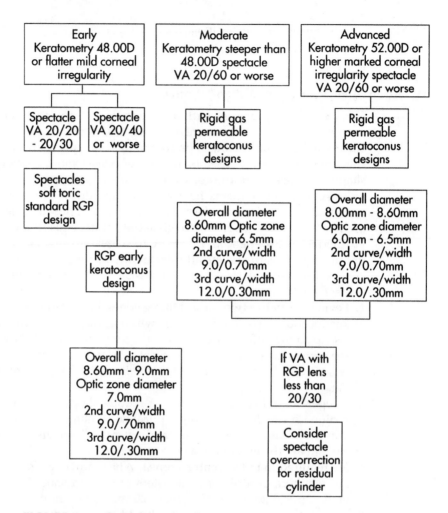

FIGURE 8-1 Guidelines for the management of keratoconus using rigid gas-permeable (RGP) contact lenses. (Courtesy Eye Sys® Laboratories, Houston)

careful evaluation of the fluorescein dye pattern may be used to adjust the peripheral lens design if necessary. Lenses that are fitted with a central clearance require flatter peripheral curve radii, which increases the peripheral lens lift.

4. Keratometer readings may be used to select the initial base curve radius that corresponds to the mean keratometer radius. Subsequent diagnostic lenses are chosen based on the fluorescein dye pattern. Alternatively, when available, computerized videokeratography also may be beneficial for proper lens selection, although enhanced efficiency of the fitting process via this technique has not been demonstrated.

CLINICAL PEARL

Subsequent diagnostic lenses are chosen based on the fluorescein dye pattern. Alternatively, when available, computerized videokeratography also may be beneficial for proper lens selection.

In the event of a consistently unstable lens fit and poor visual acuity, alternative lens designs may be considered. Residual astigmatism should be considered if there is poor visual acuity. Spectacle correction over the contact lens is often necessary for maximal visual performance in moderate to advanced keratoconus. A consistent unstable lens fit may often be improved with larger overall diameters. Central-touch base curve/cornea fitting relationships usually result. A piggyback lens system may be considered in the event of an unstable or uncomfortable lens fit. The Sofperm lens, which has a soft periphery and a rigid optical portion, may on occasion offer some patients a more stable fit with enhanced comfort. Recent introduction of steeper P.A.R. in the Sofperm design should enhance success with this unique design.

• Case Three: Penetrating Keratoplasty/Anisometropic Regular Astigmatism

I. Subjective Data

A 32-year-old man sustained a finger jab to the right cornea while playing basketball. A penetrating keratoplasty was performed 8 weeks before his examination to remove scar tissue in the visual axis. The postoperative course was uncomplicated except for graft astigmatism and anisometropia. He had worn spherical soft contact lenses without problems during the previous 10 years.

II. Objective Data

Preoperative spectacle correction

OD: −1.00 −0.50 × 165
OS: −1.75 DS

Visual acuity without correction

OD: 20/400
OS: 20/300

Keratometry

OD: 44.00 @ 165; 50.00 @ 075 (smooth mires)
OS: 42.25 @ 090; 42.75 @ 180 (smooth mires)

Manifest refraction

OD: −3.00 −5.50 × 170 (20/20)
OS: −1.50 −0.75 × 085 (20/20)

Biomicroscopy

The right eye had a clear graft with a running suture in place.

Trial frame

The above prescription was demonstrated via a trial frame. He sensed a feeling of pulling while wearing the full correction. When the cylindrical power was reduced by one third, his visual acuity decreased 2 lines.

Contact lens dispensing

A custom soft toric contact lens was dispensed having the following parameters:

PAR	Power	Diameter
8.9 mm	−3.00 −4.75 × 170	15.0 mm

Visual acuity with contact lens

OD: 20/20

The lens fit was excellent, although some (minimal) blink-induced movement was present, and less than 5° of counterclockwise rotation occurred. He continued to wear a spherical soft contact lens on the uninjured left eye.

Follow-up 2 weeks after dispensing

He was quite satisfied with the quality of his vision and comfort of the contact lens. However, the lens continued to show only a trace of blink-induced movement. Fine-vessel ingrowth was noted along the suture bites from 4 to 6 o'clock (Plate 17). Lens wear was discontinued while a flatter PAR lens (9.2 mm) was ordered.

Follow-up 6 weeks after dispensing

Visual acuity and lens comfort were excellent. The graft remained clear without neovascularization. He was instructed to remove the contact lens after no more than 14 hours of wear. A follow-up appointment was scheduled for 6 months.

III. Assessment/Plan

Despite an excellent surgical result, with a clear cornea and no graft rejection, this patient required correction of the resultant refractive error. Significant anisometropia and graft astigmatism were present. His response while wearing the required correction in a trial frame suggested that adaptation to spectacles would be unlikely. Therefore a custom toric soft contact lens was utilized.

The technique for fitting such a lens is as follows:
A diagnostic lens is ordered with powers that correspond to the *vertex corrected spectacle prescription* (Fig. 8-2). Such custom lenses are available from various manufacturers—Coastvision, Kontur, Optech, Sunsoft, and Westcon. They usually have large overall diameters (at least 15 mm) with a posterior apical radius of 8.8 to 9.0 mm. The initial lens ordered is considered the diagnostic lens. Adjustments of its fit and/or power may be made based on movement, visual acuity, and lens rotation (the LARS principle [left add, right subtract] applies). Because thick lens profiles are usually present, generous lens movement is desired to reduce hypoxia, which is probably an important factor leading to neovascularization.

IV. Alternative Management Plan/Summary

Contemporary techniques for penetrating keratoplasty result in high rates of success if based on graft clarity and a low incidence of graft failure. However, refractive error following penetrating keratoplasty should be anticipated. Therefore optical correction in the form of either spectacles or contact lenses is the rule. The appropriate form of optical correction is based on the presentation of each case. Specific criteria to consider include best corrected visual acuities, degree of anisometropia, quality of the graft surface topography, and probability of success with contact lenses (Fig. 8-3).

In general, persons above 55 years of age without a history of contact lens wear are less successful wearing contact lenses than those who are younger. In the event that spectacles and contact lenses do not solve a patient's visual needs, refractive surgical procedures (such as radial keratotomy combined with astigmatic keratotomy if necessary) may be indicated, although these procedures may be associated with subsequent graft rejection.

• Case Four: Penetrating Keratoplasty/Irregular Astigmatism

I. Subjective Data

A 57-year-old woman with a history of nuclear sclerotic cataract and Fuch's endothelial dystrophy was 4 months post–penetrating keratoplasty/extracapsular cataract extraction with posterior chamber implant in the right eye when she became disturbed that her vision was "no different from before the operation." The postoperative period was complicated by graft rejection at 2 months that responded well to aggressive immunosuppressive therapy. Visual acuity in her left eye was limited by a cataract and early corneal edema. Her

In **hyperopic** astigmatism the astigmatic correction
required at the cornea will be *greater* than that
required in the spectacle plane. Example:

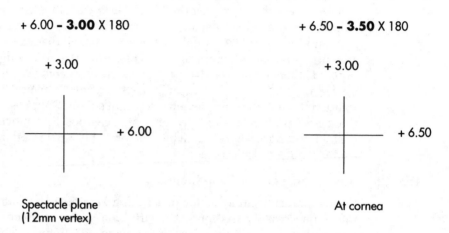

+ 6.00 - **3.00** X 180   + 6.50 - **3.50** X 180

+ 3.00   + 3.00

+ 6.00   + 6.50

Spectacle plane   At cornea
(12mm vertex)

In **myopic** astigmatism the astigmatic correction
required at the cornea will be *less* than that
required in the spectacle plane. Example:

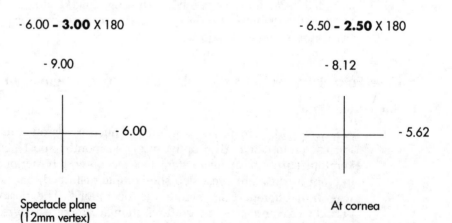

- 6.00 - **3.00** X 180   - 6.50 - **2.50** X 180

- 9.00   - 8.12

- 6.00   - 5.62

Spectacle plane   At cornea
(12mm vertex)

FIGURE 8-2 Effect of a change in vertex distance on the required
astigmatic correction.

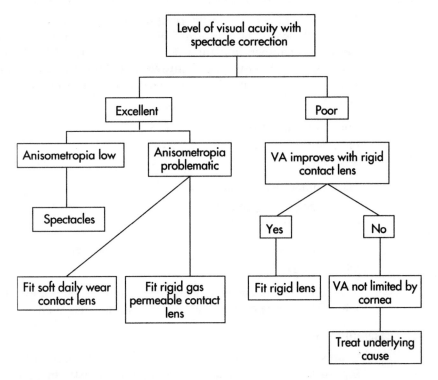

FIGURE 8-3 Options for optical correction after penetrating keratoplasty.

medications included artificial tears qid and prednisolone acetate 1% qd OD.

II. Objective Data

Visual acuity without correction

OD: 20/200   (pinhole 20/40)
OS: 20/100   (pinhole 20/60)

Manifest refraction

OD: 5.00 –2.00 × 135 (20/100)
OS: +0.75 –1.25 × 100 (20/60)

Distorted retinoscopy reflex OU

Keratometry

OD: 47.00 @ 150; 48.50 @ 60 (distorted and irregular mires)
OS: 41.50 DS (smooth mires)

Biomicroscopy

The 7.5 mm graft in the *right eye* was mostly clear except for posterior stromal haze from 5 to 7 o'clock along with three folds at the level of

Descemet's membrane in the central graft. The anterior chamber was deep and clear. The iris formed a round pupil without synechiae. A posterior chamber implant was in place. In the *left eye* numerous endothelial guttata were present without clinically significant epithelial or stromal edema. A mixed nuclear sclerotic and cortical cataract was observed.

Potential acuity meter

OD: 20/25
OS: 20/30

Hard contact lens parameters

	BCR	OAD/OZD	Power
OD:	7.03 mm	9.0/7.0 mm	−3.00 D

Overrefraction

OD: −1.50 D   (20/25)

The contact lens centered well with 2 mm of blink-induced movement. Noticeable central graft touch was also observed.

III. Assessment/Plan

Graft surface irregularities are often the most important factors limiting visual acuity after a penetrating keratoplasty. In such cases the quality of vision through the optimum spectacle prescription is disappointing. Typically special testing (such as potential acuity) will predict a level of vision far better than that obtained with spectacles. Furthermore, as in the above case, visual acuity through a rigid contact lens is usually improved over that obtained with spectacles. Therefore an RGP contact lens was the recommended optical correction for this patient. Because a relatively steep graft was present, the interpalpebral fitting philosophy with a PAR steeper than "K" was considered (Plate 18 and Fig. 8-4). Spectacles were prescribed to be worn over the contact lens for a near bifocal correction. Surgery for the left eye was planned once maximal and stable optical rehabilitation had been obtained for the right eye.

IV. Alternative Management Plan/Summary

Irregular astigmatism (which cannot be neutralized by spectacle lenses) may result from various optical conditions.

First, it may occur when the major refractive meridians are not "orthogonal" (that is, the maximum and minimum powers are separated by an angle ≠ 90°). Such situations may result from IOL malposition, a decentered or tilted graft, or unequal suture tension. Doubling the keratometer mires along with scissors motion during retinoscopy is present. Analysis of Placido's rings and/or computer

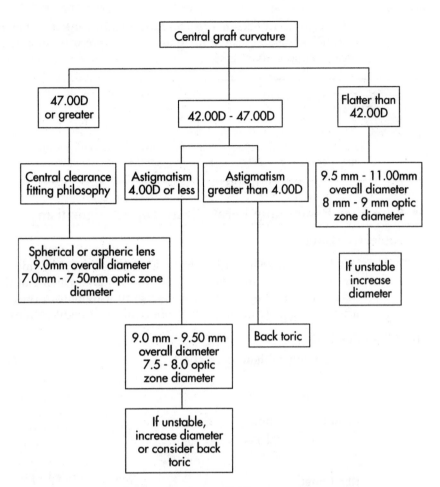

FIGURE 8-4 Guidelines for fitting RGP contact lenses after penetrating keratoplasty.

assisted videokeratography may show a decentered central ring (Plate 19). If the graft is determined to be the source of such irregularities, an RGP lens is indicated. Irregular astigmatism that is the result of a malpositioned intraocular lens, however, (contrary thought) will not be neutralized by a contact lens.

A second and more common source of irregular astigmatism, particularly in patients over 50 years of age, is tear film and surface abnormalities. The keratometer mires may be quite distorted with an unclear endpoint. The retinoscopy reflex is often dim and not well defined. Such astigmatism may result from keratoconjunctivitis sicca or from malposition of the graft/host interface, the latter due to an asymmetrical healing response in some patients. Early fitting of RGP lenses (near the 3-month postoperative period) may decrease the severity of graft irregularities and astigmatism. Alternatively, tincture of time may be indicated for patients who are unable or reluctant to wear a rigid contact lens.

CLINICAL PEARL

Such astigmatism may result from keratoconjunctivitis sicca or from malposition of the graft/host interface, the latter due to an asymmetrical healing response in some patients. Early fitting of RGP lenses (near the 3-month postoperative period) may decrease the severity of graft irregularities and astigmatism.

• Case Five: Penetrating Keratoplasty/High Astigmatism

I. Subjective Data

A 49-year-old man with a history of penetrating trauma who had received a penetrating keratoplasty for residual scarring at the visual axis of the right eye had significant graft astigmatism present 1 year after the transplant. He was unable to drive at night because of glare.

II. Objective Data

Visual acuity without correction

OD: 20/100
OS: 20/25

Manifest refraction

OD: 1.00 −6.00 × 135   (20/30)
OS: +0.50 −0.75 × 100   (20/20)

Keratometry

OD: 45.00 @ 140; 51.50 @ 50   (minimal distortion)
OS: 43.50 DS   (smooth mires)

Biomicroscopy

In the right eye the graft was clear. Sutures had been removed previously. In the left eye all structures were free of pathology.

Hard contact lens refraction

BCR	OAD/OZD	Power
48.00 D (7.03 mm)	9.0/7.0 mm	−3.00 D

Visual acuity

20/20−

The visual acuity was variable because of excessive lens movement. Approximately 90% of the time the lens was positioned on the inferior third of the cornea.

III. Assessment/Plan

The cause of this patient's visual loss was twofold. First, similar to Case Three, a high degree of graft astigmatism was present. However, second, there were surface irregularities that further decreased the best potential visual acuity. This was demonstrated by the distorted keratometer mires, along with the improved visual acuity that occurred with a diagnostic hard contact lens overrefraction. Thus maximum vision performance was made possible with a rigid contact lens.

To obtain a stable RGP contact lens fit for patients who have high astigmatism following penetrating keratoplasty, a back toric and/or bitoric lens design should be considered. A good initial design is a lens having a back corneal toricity equal to 75% of the graft astigmatism. The flatter PAR should then approximately align with the flatter corneal meridian.

I prefer bitoric designs that have a *spherical power effect* so the blink-induced lens torsional movements do not reduce visual acuity. Clinicians attempting to fit such lenses will be well served by an SPE bitoric diagnostic fitting set (see box).

IV. Alternative Management Plan/Summary

This relatively young patient was troubled by a high, slightly irregular, graft astigmatism. Before the injury, he had been accustomed to excellent uncorrected visual acuity in each eye. Such patients are usually very determined to maximize their visual acuity following trauma. Clinicians should strive for a level of vision equal to or better than that in the uninjured eye so the patient will have an incentive to proceed with contact lens correction. This is particularly important if the injured eye was the patient's habitually dominant eye.

Graft astigmatism greater than 4 D is considered high and likely to result in an unstable lens fit with spherical RGP lens designs.

Guidelines for fitting back-surface toric and bitoric contact lenses

Spherical power effect (SPE) diagnostic lenses are recommended (3 to 4 D toric).
Toricity in the contact lens should equal two thirds to three fourths that in the corneal cylinder.
Fit the flat meridian either on "K" or 0.50 D flatter than "K."
Order an SPE design if possible (depending on visual acuity).
If the fit is unstable, increase the diameter and/or back toricity.

Exceptions to this trend include grafts with a small central zone of astigmatism (such as occurs with relatively steep grafts often associated with the double running suture technique). If the major power meridians measured by keratometry are greater than 48.00 D, spherical RGP lens designs may prove to be stable when a central clearance/ fitting relationship is utilized.

CLINICAL PEARL

If the major power meridians measured by keratometry are greater than 48.00 D, spherical RGP lens designs may prove to be stable when a central clearance/fitting relationship is utilized.

Astigmatism in grafts flatter than 48.00 D usually manifests over a larger chord diameter. Although it is prudent to use a spherical design if possible, bitoric lenses are usually more comfortable and provide a more stable fit for high astigmatism occurring in a relatively flat graft.

• Case Six: Pellucid Degeneration

I. Subjective Data

A 48-year-old woman with no history of contact lens wear complained of blurred vision in her right eye. She had been wearing spectacles since age 13, and was diagnosed with pellucid marginal degeneration 5 years before her most recent visit.

II. Objective Data

Visual acuity with spectacles

OD: 20/60
OS: 20/30

Habitual spectacle correction

OD: −2.00 −3.50 × 65
OS: −1.75 −4.00 × 80

Manifest refraction

OD: −3.00 −6.50 × 60 (20/40)   (pinhole 20/25)
OS: −2.25 −4.50 × 75 (20/25−)

Keratometry

OD: 45.00 @ 180; 40.00 @ 090 (irregular mires)
OS: 45.00 @ 180; 41.00 @ 090 (irregular mires)

Biomicroscopy

An area of marked thinning (> 50%) was observed within the inferior fourth of both corneas, which were otherwise clear.

Photokeratoscopy

Steepening along the inferior hemimeridian was noted, with marked flattening along the superior hemimeridian (OD > OS) (Plate 20). An RGP contact lens with the following parameters was placed on the right eye:

BCR	OAD/OZD	Power
40.00 (8.43 mm)	9.6/8.0 mm	−3.00 D

Visual acuity

20/25

The fit was mostly inferior, with an inferior edge standoff.

III. Assessment/Plan

This patient was motivated to improve her vision if at all possible. Therefore a large-diameter lens was ordered in parameters similar to those of the above diagnostic lens.

IV. Alternative Management Plan/ Summary

Pellucid degeneration is characterized by marked thinning on the inferior fourth of the cornea that results in a flattened superior vertical profile with subsequent against-the-rule astigmatism. It is quite rare. Some authors consider it to be an atypical form of keratoconus. However, the thinning is more peripheral than that found in typical keratoconus. Therefore curvature differences between the superior and inferior cornea of 10 to 15 D or more are common. Success with RGP lenses in this patient population is lower than that obtained with typical keratoconus. The lenses typically must be relatively large, with a base curve radius that aligns on the superior half of the cornea, and thus have a marked inferior edge lift that may prove to be uncomfortable.

Many patients with pellucid degeneration do well wearing spectacles that incorporate a high cylindrical correction. Penetrating keratoplasty is postponed until all spectacle and contact lens options have proven unsuccessful. The procedure is less predictable than that for keratoconus because the thinning is more peripheral.

• Case Seven: Post–Refractive Surgery

I. Subject Data

A 35-year-old myopic high school basketball coach underwent radial keratotomy of the right eye in June 1991 and the left eye in June 1992.

An eight-incision technique (3.5 mm optical zone) was utilized on the right eye, and a four-incision technique (3.5 mm optical zone) on the left. He desired the best corrected visual acuity possible while working with his players.

II. Objective Data

Visual acuity without correction

OD: 20/40
OS: 20/30

Preoperative manifest refraction

OD: −4.50 −1.00 × 170 (20/15)
OS: −4.00 −0.75 × 180 (20/15)

Keratometry

OD: 43.50 @ 180; 44.25 @ 090
OS: −43.00 DS (smooth mires)

Postoperative manifest refraction

OD: +1.00 −0.75 × 150 (20/25)
OS: −0.75 −0.75 × 160 (20/20)

Keratometry

OD: 39.50 @ 180; 40.25 @ 090 (slightly irregular mires)
OS: 40 DS (smooth mires)

Habitual spectacle correction

OD: +1.25 −0.75 × 150
OS: −0.75 −1.00 × 170

Biomicroscopy

In the right eye eight radial incisions extending to the limbus were present. Three were noted to extend into the visual axis on the temporal pupillary margin. In the left eye four radial incisions were present that spared the limbus, ending approximately 1 mm in front of it. A uniform 3.5 mm optical zone was allowed to remain.

III. Assessment/Plan

This patient demonstrated two of the numerous outcomes following radial keratotomy. The first procedure, performed on his right eye, resulted in overcorrection of the myopia. The second procedure, on the left eye, involved fewer incisions and resulted in the more desirable outcome of undercorrection. Furthermore, in addition to a greater reduction in myopia for the right eye, surface irregularities were present that was probably due to in an asymmetrical incision length. The patient was an emerging presbyope, and thus surgical overcorrection in the right eye was problematical. It was recommended therefore that he be fitted with a contact lens in the right eye. An RGP lens was selected to neutralize surface irregularities. A soft contact lens was not considered because the incisions that extended to the limbus probably would have predisposed the cornea to neovascularization. The lens diameter and base curve radii were chosen to align with the transition between a flat central zone and the steeper midperiphery (Plate 21).

In most cases this design shows a dye pattern that is steep over the central flat cornea. If a stable lens fit is not possible, designs incorporating secondary curves that are steeper than the base curves can be obtained (RK-Bridge by Conforma, Norfolk Va, and O-K Lens by Contex, Sherman Oaks Calif). These allow for a flatter PAR without compromising the stability of fit.

IV. Alternative Management Plan/Summary

When contact lenses are required after a refractive surgical procedure such as radial keratotomy, clinicians should consider the probability that this circumstance was unplanned. Careful preoperative counseling will often prepare patients for such an occurrence and thereby reduce their disappointment if contact lenses are indicated after the procedure. Rigid gas-permeable (RGP) contact lenses are indicated for irregular astigmatism and are preferred after procedures in which the incisions extend to the limbus. Neovascularization of the incisions is likely when soft contact lenses are worn following this technique. In the above case a soft contact lens would be an option for the left eye, which had only four cuts with shorter incisions that did not extend to the limbus.

Summary

Optical rehabilitation for patients with corneal disease or following surgery is both rewarding and challenging for clinicians. Recent advances in contact lens material and design technology provide the fitter excellent alternatives for enhancing vision performance in this unique patient population. To maximize patient satisfaction and quality of vision, successful clinicians will utilize their imagination along with the numerous options for correction.

9

Management of Contact Lens–Induced Complications

Robert M. Grohe
Neelu K. Hira

Routine contact lens wear can be safe and uneventful. However, a wide range of complications may also occur, induced by or related to either daily or extended contact lens wear. Complications can be created by factors such as lens materials, solution systems, improper eye/lens design relationships, or simply noncompliance. Since the practitioner exerts direct control over all these factors except noncompliance, it is important to be aware of specific complications induced by or related to certain lens types and/or solutions.

Complications arising from patient noncompliance are elusive and hard to correct, since they frequently are the product of previous contact lens experiences.[16] Therefore, it is vital that practitioners and their contact lens assistants seek out, identify, and remedy (through reeducation) problem areas of noncompliance—such as confusion over solution use, mishandling, self-discontinuation of recommended care regimens, and brand substitution of solutions. This chapter will review examples of contact lens induced or related complications that are common or unique to clinical practice. Each case will be followed by a discussion of alternative options in managing clinically challenging examples.

• Case One: Contact Lens–Induced Abrasions

I. Subjective Data

A 64-year-old man with a 4-year history of bilateral aphakia and rigid gas-permeable (RGP) lens wear urgently called with a complaint of sudden pain upon lens insertion in the right eye. He had a contact lens handling history that was noteworthy for aggressive and reckless insertion techniques despite numerous attempts to alter via reeducation, reminders, and retraining.

II. Objective Data

Visual acuity

OD: 20/200
OS: 20/25

Overrefraction

OD: No improvement
OS: −0.25 (20/20)

Current contact lenses

		BCR*	BVP	OAD/OZD	
OD:	Equalens	7.93 mm	+18.50 D	9.8/8.0 mm	(−) lenticular
OS:	Equalens	7.85	+20.00 D	9.8/8.0 mm	(−) lenticular

Current spectacle prescription

OD: +16.00 −1.00 × 180   (20/200)
OS: +18.25 −0.50 × 165   (20/30)

Manifest refraction

OD: +15.50 −0.75 × 180   (20/200)
OS: +18.25 −0.75 × 167   (20/25)

Keratometry

OD: 42.00 @ 165; 43.00 @ 075   (gross mire distortion)
OS: 42.12 @ 165; 42.75 @ 075   (smooth mires)

Slit-lamp examination

The right contact lens had been removed at home, and the cornea had a 1.25 × 3.0 mm central abrasion with a deep uptake of fluorescein (Plate 22). The left RGP lens was positioned centrally, with 3 mm of movement present after the blink. There was mild nasal and temporal dustlike arcuate staining. The patient was advised to discontinue wearing the right lens and was treated with Polytrim qid, along with

---

*BCR, base curve radius; BVP, back vertex power; OAD, overall diameter; OZD optical zone diameter.

a bandage soft contact lens to minimize eye discomfort. He persisted in rubbing the closed right eye with his knuckles, however, even after repeated explanations, admonitions, and physical restraint. He was instructed to return the next day but did not appear until 3 days later, at which time (despite office protests) he stated that he wished to be refracted.

Manifest refraction

OD: +16.00 – 0.75 × 180   (20/40)
OS: +18.25 – 0.50 × 167   (20/25)

Keratometry

OD: 42.00 @ 180; 42.62 @ 090   (mild mire distortion)
OS: 42.00 @ 165; 42.75 @ 075   (smooth mires)

Slit-lamp examination

The right eye had a remarkably smaller abraded area of approximately 0.20 mm in a circular central pattern. He was advised to continue not wearing the right contact lens for 4 more days. Polytrim was decreased to tid.

At the next follow-up visit he presented with the following:

Manifest refraction

OD: +16.25 –1.00 × 180   (20/25)
OS: +18.25 –0.50 × 167   (20/25)

Keratometry

OD: 42.12 @ 180; 42.75 @ 090   (smooth mires)
OS: 42.00 @ 165; 42.62 @ 075   (smooth mires)

Lens inspection

Both lenses had intact and smooth edges with stable parameters.

Biomicroscopy

The right cornea was now completely healed, without any staining or anterior chamber reaction. Polytrim was discontinued, and the patient advised to return to right contact lens wear beginning with 4 to 6 hours the first day and increasing by 1 to 2 hours per day until he was able to resume all-day wearing.

At the third follow-up visit (1 month after the initial abrasion) he presented with

Visual acuity wearing RGPs

OD: 20/20-3
OS: 20/20-2
OU: 20/20-1

Keratometry

OD: 41.87 @ 180; 42.62 @ 090   (smooth mires)
OS: 41.75 @ 180; 42.50 @ 090   (smooth mires)

Slit-lamp examination

No central corneal staining was present in either eye. He was now wearing the RGPs a total of 16 hours per day but did admit to continued insertion techniques that were more aggressive than desirable.

III. Assessment/Plan

This patient was victimized by his reckless lens handling habits and a tendency for unclipped fingernails. With greater attention to personal hygiene and handling techniques, he has subsequently avoided any further abrasion incidents. The office staff continues to remind him at each office visit of the importance of lens handling. In this instance the consequence of lens mishandling (abrasion) reinforced the urge to change habits. However, not all patients can be assumed to react in a similar manner. Clinicians should expect regression unless continued patient contact and reinforcement of instructions prove otherwise.

IV. Alternative Management Plan/Summary

Abrasions can become a gateway for pathogens, inflammation, infections, and ultimately ulcers. Contact lens–induced abrasions may be caused by a variety of factors, as summarized in the box. After ruling out physical defects during lens inspection, practitioners must turn to a careful review of the handling practices used by the patient. Due to feelings of embarrassment or shame, patients may not always be eager to discuss and/or reveal self-induced causes of abrasions. Diplomacy and patience will assist in determining most circumstances. However, before any lens wear is resumed, there must always be complete corneal healing. An incompletely healed cornea is a poor barrier to infection, inflammation, or ulceration.

• Case Two: Infiltrates with Soft Contact Lenses

I. Subjective Data

A 32-year-old woman presented with a 2-day history of irritation in her right eye, which was slightly red. She also stated that she had an increased awareness of fluorescent lights and, in addition, had noticed a "funny white spot on the colored part" of her right cornea. She was a daily-wear, 2-week disposable, soft contact lens wearer who sometimes got "confused" about the actual length of time she had been wearing a particular pair of lenses; and there had also been, she admitted, a tendency to forget to change her disinfection solution every day.

Factors Contributing to Abrasions with Contact Lens Wear

Lens design
  Poor blending
  Sharp edges
Lens edge defects
  Serrated
  Chipped
  Fragmented
Chemical agents
  Preservative(s)
  Disinfection systems
  Surfactant cleaners
  Enzyme cleaners
  Cosmetics
Foreign bodies
Environmental vapors
Patient mishandling
  Aggressive insertion
  Long fingernails
  Eye rubbing with lens on the eye

II. Objective Data

Visual acuity

OD: 20/40
OS: 20/20

Overrefraction

OD: No improvement
OS: Plano (20/20)

Current contact lens specifications

	Brand	BCR	OAD	Power
OD:	Seequence II	8.7 mm	14.0 mm	−3.00 D
OS:	Seequence II	8.7 mm	14.0 mm	−2.75 D

Current spectacle prescription

OD: −3.00 DS (20/20)
OS: −2.75 DS (20/20)

Manifest refraction

OD: −3.00 DS (20/20)
OS: −2.75 DS (20/20)

Keratometry

OD: 42.50 @ 180; 42.87 @ 090 (slight mire distortion)
OS: 42.87 @ 180; 43.00 @ 090 (smooth mires)

Biomicroscopy

The right conjunctiva was moderately injected in the temporal globe, and the right cornea had a 1.5 mm circular subepithelial infiltrate adjacent to the limbus at 9 o'clock with mild epithelial elevation and an overlying superficial punctate keratitis. Fluorescein staining did not extend beyond the perimeter of the infiltrate. Some flare and cells were present in the anterior chamber. The left eye appeared to be quiet and uninvolved. She was advised to discontinue all contact lens wear. Cyclopentolate (Cyclogyl 1%) and a combination steroid-antibacterial drop (Tobradex) qid were prescribed. Cultures were not taken because of the absence of any ulcerlike lesion. She was instructed to return the following day but was unable to do so. Two days later she presented with the following:

Visual acuity wearing spectacles

OD: 20/25
OS: 20/20

Keratometry

OD: 42.50 @ 180; 42.62 @ 090   (smooth mires)
OS: 42.87 @ 180; 43.12 @ 090   (smooth mires)

Biomicroscopy

The right cornea had a 0.5 mm diffuse subepithelial infiltrate without any vascularization whose density had significantly decreased. There was no sign of any anterior chamber reaction. The left eye was quiet. She was instructed to continue wearing spectacles and to avoid all contact lens wear. The cycloplegic was eliminated, and the Tobradex continued qid for 4 days and then tid for 7 days. She was asked to return in 10 days. Eleven days later she presented with

Visual acuity wearing spectacles

OD: 20/20
OS: 20/20

Keratometry

OD: 42.37 @ 180; 42.75 @ 090   (smooth mires)
OS: 42.75 @ 180; 43.00 @ 090   (smooth mires)

Manifest refraction

OD: −3.00 DS   (20/20)
OS: −2.75 DS   (20/20)

The right cornea was now clear and free of any fluorescein staining. The right anterior chamber was deep and quiet. The left eye was quiet and normal. She was instructed to continue tapering the Tobradex, using it bid for 7 days and then qd for 7 more days, and was given fresh disinfecting solution and a new lens case.

III. Assessment/Plan

This patient was fortunate not to have developed a corneal ulcer. The symptoms prompted her to seek care. However, not all subepithelial infiltrates will cause dramatic symptoms. Clinicians should always remain sensitive to patient comments about pain, photophobia, or "white spots on the eye" noted during self-examination. These are typically significant and require immediate attention. Even if the ultimate clinical outcome is unremarkable, once the patient arrives at the office it is imperative that contact lens clinicians err on the conservative side of follow-up care.

CLINICAL PEARL

Clinicians should always remain sensitive to patient comments about pain, photophobia, or "white spots on the eye" noted during self-examination.

Not all subepithelial infiltrates will cause an anterior chamber reaction. Indeed, an iritis often accompanies more serious conditions (such as corneal ulcers).[7] Therefore a cycloplegic was selected in this case to quickly quiet the anterior chamber and reduce any secondary pain from ciliary spasm. Although several types of combination drugs are available, Tobradex was chosen for its ability to stabilize mild inflammatory lesions, such as the subepithelial infiltrate noted in this case.

IV. Alternative Management Plan/Summary

A subepithelial infiltrate can deteriorate into an erosion or, even worse, an ulcer. Many factors are contributory—from patient inattention to friction when a hydrogel lens surface or the edge of an RGP rubs the eye. Further complicating the condition is the potential for microbiological contamination, leading to a combined infection, inflammation, and/or ulcer. Therefore clinicians need to astutely discriminate between subepithelial infiltrates and corneal ulcers. An infiltrate is shown in Plate 23.

A summary of the differential diagnosis for sterile infiltrates versus infected ulcers has been suggested by Stein et al.[15] and is given in Table 9-1. The key factors to monitor are discomfort, discharge,

TABLE 9-1

Signs and Symptoms: Sterile Infiltrates Versus Infected Ulcers

	Sterile Infiltrate	Infected Ulcer
Discomfort	Mild to moderate	Moderate to severe
Discharge	Absent (100%)	Present (80%)
Lesion size	Variable (0.1 to 0.9 mm)	Greater than 2 mm
Overlying epithelial defect	None (may be superficial punctate keratitis)	Always
Anterior chamber reaction	Absent to mild	Moderate to severe
Shape of lesion	Significant if arcuate (i.e., tight lens)	Significant if ring (i.e., *Acanthamoeba*)

*Modified from Stein RM, et al: *Am J Ophthalmol* 105:632-636, 1988.

lesion size, an overlying epithelial defect, an anterior chamber reaction, and the shape of the lesion. All these factors worsen and/or increase with corneal ulcers. Additionally, it has been observed that the location of a corneal lesion may be an indicator of severity, with sterile infiltrates localized more in the periphery and infected ulcers seeming to occur more in the center or midperiphery.

CLINICAL PEARL

The key factors to monitor are discomfort, discharge, lesion size, an overlying epithelial defect, an anterior chamber reaction, and the shape of the lesion.

Treatment utilized for sterile infiltrates versus infected ulcers varies significantly and is very time dependent. Thus it is vital in a differential diagnosis to define the specific condition so treatment can be customized to it. Of greater urgency is treatment for corneal ulcers, which may require immediate hospitalization if the condition is nonresponsive to initial treatment. A summary of the comparative treatments used for sterile infiltrates and corneal ulcers is given in the box. Controversy exists concerning the use of corticosteroids in ulcer cases because of *Pseudomonas* proliferating into an epithelium that is not intact.[10] Except in extreme circumstances, such as potential corneal perforation, patching is contraindicated in either condition.[10]

We and others[2] recommend the following clinical data as beneficial in monitoring any suspected corneal lesion:

1. Patient perception of pain and photophobia
2. Drawing of area and number of subepithelial infiltrates
3. Drawing of size and depth of the ulcer
4. Drawing of the epithelial defect

Comparative Treatment Regimens

Sterile Infiltrates	Ulcers
Discontinue all contact lens wear	Discontinue all contact lens wear
Antibiotics	Culture/sensitivity studies*
Taper topical steroids	Broad-spectrum fortified
qid × 7 days	antibiotics q30min
bid × 7 days	Aminoglycosides (Tobramycin)
bid × 7 days	Cephalosporins (Cefazolin)
qd × 7 days	Cycloplegics (homatropine 2% bid)
Close follow-up	Oral analgesics
	Return *stat* if
	Vision decreases
	Pain increases
	If nonresponsive or worsening
	Reculture 48 hr after treatment
	Reculture q24h until negative
	If no improvement, promptly
	refer out

*Immediate hospitalization for treatment with fortified antibiotics may be necessary.

---

5. Drawing of surrounding stromal edema
6. Distance from center of cornea
7. Anterior chamber reaction
8. Amount/color/consistency of discharge
9. Scleral involvement
10. R/O perforation

An epithelial defect is the most common factor inducing a microbial keratitis. Thus an abrasion, epithelial bulla, erosion, or foreign body can induce a corneal ulcer. Since both immunological and infectious infiltrates occur at the limbus,[2] contact lens practitioners need to utilize a lens design that minimizes any potential friction in the corneal periphery or the limbus.

• Case Three: Vascularization with RGPs

I. Subjective Data

A 36-year-old woman was referred by an eye care practitioner for a possible RGP refitting due to bilateral vessel growth into the cornea. She had previously worn PMMA contact lenses for 16 years and was currently wearing RGPs (5 years). The only symptom was a mild redness apparent to her and her friends during her customary 14 hours of lens wear each day. She also reported that her lenses always "dropped down" on her eyes when she looked into a mirror while applying makeup.

II. Objective Data

Visual acuity

OD: 20/25
OS: 20/25

Overrefraction

OD: −0.50 D   (20/20)
OS: −0.50 D   (20/20)

Current contact lens prescription

		BCR	Power	OAD/OZD	CT
OD:	Boston II (single-cut design)	7.52 mm	−5.00 D	8.8/8.0 mm	0.16 mm
OS:	Boston II (single-cut design)	7.54 mm	−4.50 D	8.8/8.0 mm	0.16 mm

Current spectacle prescription

OD: −4.75   −0.50 × 180
OS: −4.00   −0.75 × 165

Manifest refraction

OD: −4.50   −0.75 × 180 (20/20)
OS: −4.25   −0.50 × 170 (20/20)

Keratometry

OD: 44.00 @ 180; 44.50 @ 90 (smooth mires)
OS: 44.25 @ 170; 44.62 @ 80 (smooth mires)

Biomicroscopy

With both contact lenses on the eyes there was marked bilateral inferior decentration. Fluorescein showed moderate arcuate midperipheral and central clearance with minimal peripheral edge clearance. There was also inferior edge clearance across the limbus with 0.5 mm overlap onto the inferior conjunctiva. When the lenses were removed, both eyes revealed moderate nasal and temporal arcuate staining in areas just adjacent to where the superior lens edges were positioned after lens decentration with the blink. There was a light semilinear central corneal stain. Bilateral diffuse temporal and nasal conjunctival injection was also present. Superficial corneal vascularization into the corneas measuring 2.5 mm in width extended 2 mm into the right temporal cornea, 2 mm across, and 2 mm into the left nasal cornea (Plate 24).

The patient was informed of this vascular growth into both corneas and that it was probably induced by several factors—including her long years of PMMA wear and her currently decentered RGP lenses. She was advised that differently designed RGP lenses, positioned superiorly and in a higher-DK material, might allow for a moderate decrease in her vessel growth and persistent conjunctival injection. New lenses were ordered with an alignment design in the Boston Equalens material.

At a follow-up visit 2 weeks later she presented with the following:

Visual acuity wearing the new RGPs

OD: 20/20
OS: 20/20

The Boston Equalens material was in a lenticular design with heavy blends.

OD: 7.69   −4.00   9.2/7.6   0.4/9.5   0.4/11.5 mm   0.16
OS: 7.71   −3.75   9.2/7.6   0.4/9.5   0.4/11.5 mm   0.16

The lenses were designed in an apical clearance fashion with a flatter central base curve/cornea relationship and a smaller optical zone. The edge clearance was greater than in the originally worn lenses.

Keratometry

OD: 44.00 @ 180; 44.62 @ 090
OS: 44.12 @ 170; 44.75 @ 080

Biomicroscopy

The RGPs centered superiorly on each eye, with 3 mm of lens movement after the blink. Fluorescein revealed a mild apical alignment with moderate edge clearance. The previous location and the amount of staining, vascularization, and injection were the same. Since the patient had continued to wear her old RGPs 14 hours per day, she was instructed to continue wearing the new lenses for the same number of hours. She was also informed that vessel growth would be slow in regressing and that her next office visit should be in 4 weeks. She returned 1 month later showing

Visual acuity with the new RGPs

OD: 20/20
OS: 20/20

Keratometry

OD: 44.12 @ 180; 44.62 @ 090   (smooth mires)
OS: 44.00 @ 170; 44.62 @ 080   (smooth mires)

Biomicroscopy

With the RGPs on, there was bilateral superior lens positioning with 2 mm of movement on the blink. Fluorescein revealed mild apical clearance with a moderate edge lift. It also showed a dramatic decrease in the previous juxtapositional lateral staining, with regression of all central superficial punctate keratitis. The right cornea had an almost undetectable amount of blood present within a diffuse and barely visible temporal ghost vessel network. The left cornea had no blood present within a poorly visualized 1.0 mm ghost vessel network extending from the limbus into the nasal cornea. Bilateral conjunctival lateral injection was subtle and barely visualized. The patient was informed of her marked improvement in staining, vascularization, and injection. She was instructed to continue her daily-wear use only after the RGPs and to return to the office in 3 months for a follow-up evaluation.

III. Assessment/Plan

As it is for many patients, the vascularization in this case was without symptoms and thus difficult for the patient to understand or accept as serious. The use of slide photodocumentation or video footage depicting inferior lens positioning and the juxtaposition of the lens against vessel growth can be beneficial in educating such a patient and helping him or her accept the need for treatment. Since many factors contribute to or enhance rigid lens vascularization, practitioners must consider the physiological and physical changes necessary in lens refitting. This patient promptly benefited from (1) a change in lens design that provided superiorly aligned lens positioning and (2) a higher Dk material that provided better oxygenation to the central and peripheral cornea.

Although no single change in lens design or material is likely to eliminate vascularization, when all these factors are combined they can synergistically reduce vessel progression.

CLINICAL PEARL

The use of slide photodocumentation or video footage that depicts inferior lens positioning and juxtapositioning of the lens against vessel growth can be beneficial in educating a patient and helping him or her accept the need for treatment.

IV. Alternative Management Plan/Summary

Vascularization of the cornea with RGP lens wear is a relatively uncommon condition. Several reports[11,12] have been cited regarding vascularization with either PMMAs or RGPs. Because most cases are asymptomatic, it is incumbent on the practitioner to detect this complication early in its development. The major part of vascularization with RGP lenses appears to be very slow in its progression. One exception to this would be vessel growth within the incision canals of post–radial keratotomy patients, which can be somewhat faster in its progression relative to that seen in a non-operated cornea. Although vascularization alone may be asymptomatic and slow to progress, if it is also associated with or encircles a peripheral corneal infiltrate there can be rapid worsening of the condition to include pain. The combination of vascularization, epithelial defect, infiltrate, and discomfort is known as vascularized limbal keratitis or VLK[9] and requires immediate lens discontinuation with an eventual refitting after regression of the infiltrate. An alternative to RGP lens design or material upgrade is to convert to hydrogel lenses or discontinue lens wear altogether. Although this may be necessary at times, clinicians should use continual monitoring in cases of hydrogel refitting since hydrogel lens–associated vascularization can also occur.

• Case Four: Filtering Blebs and RGP Lens Wear

I. Subjective Data

A 63-year-old woman with an 11-year rigid lens history (5 years PMMA, 6 years RGP) who underwent bilateral cataract surgery for primary open-angle glaucoma experienced aphakia and a filtering bleb in her left eye. She had experienced recent bouts of left contact lens awareness and occasional sudden sharp pains in that eye. She also reported a lifelong amblyopia, greater in the left than in the right eye.

II. Objective Data

Visual acuity with RGPs

OD: 20/40
OS: 20/50

Overrefraction

OD: +0.25 D (20/30)
OS: No improvement

Current RGP prescription

	Design	BCR	Power	OAD/OZD	CT
OD:	Boston II, (–) lenticular	7.20 mm	+14.50 D	9.0/7.8 mm	0.30 mm
OS:	Boston II, (–) lenticular	7.57 mm	6.00 D	9.0/7.8 mm	0.35 mm

Manifest refraction

OD: +5.25 –1.00 × 150   (20/30)
OS: +6.00 –.75 × 90   (20/50)

Keratometry

OD: 46.25 @ 150; 46.75 @ 060   (no inferior steepening)
OS: 44.75 @ 180; 44.25 @ 090   (no inferior steepening)

Biomicroscopy

With RGPs, the right lens was positioned centrally with less than 1 mm of movement and a low peripheral edge clearance. The left lens was positioned centrally with about 1 mm of movement and a shallow edge clearance. Bilateral fluorescein revealed mild apical clearance. Without contact lenses the right cornea clearly had no scars and a white conjunctiva. The left cornea was clear, without scars and with a small slightly lobulated filtering bleb on the superior nasal conjunctiva between 10 and 11 o'clock. The bleb appeared white and glistening, with a normal reflex and its anterior edge just beyond the limbus. No vascularization was observed. Fluorescein revealed no stain uptake at or around the bleb site. Because of intermittent lens awareness and pain in her left eye, it was decided to replace both lenses to improve lens movement and minimize possible lens encroachment on the filtering bleb.

New RGP prescription

	Design	BCR	Power	OAD/OZD
OD:	Boston Equalens, (–) lenticular	7.28 mm	+5.50 D	9.0/7.4 mm
OS:	Boston Equalens, (–) lenticular	7.62 mm	+6.25 D	8.8/7.6 mm

	SCR (W)	PCR (W)	CT
OD:	9.25(0.3 mm)	11.50(0.3 mm)	0.31 mm
OS:	9.60(0.3 mm)	11.80(0.3 mm)	0.36 mm

At the follow-up/dispensing visit 10 days later

Visual acuity with new lenses

OD: 20/30
OS: 20/50

Overrefraction

OD: No improvement
OS: No improvement

Keratometry

OD: 46.12 @ 150; 46.75 @ 060   (no inferior steepening)
OS: 44.62 @ 180; 44.12 @ 090   (no inferior steepening)

Biomicroscopy

Both lenses positioned superiorly, decentering centrally between blinks. Each had 2 to 3 mm of movement. Fluorescein revealed a mild apical clearing. No superficial punctate keratitis (SPK) was noted, although there was an absence of lens contact with the bleb in the left eye. The patient was instructed to continue normal lens wear and to return to the office in 3 months. At the next follow-up visit (9 months later) she came into the office complaining of increased irritation in her left eye when she wore the lens. This had been going on for the preceding month. She also stated that she thought she had seen a small amount of blood (diluted) in the corner of her right eye.

Visual acuity with lenses

OD: 20/30
OS: 20/50

Overrefraction

OD: No improvement
OS: No improvement

Keratometry

OD: 46.25 @ 150; 46.87 @ 060   (no inferior steepening)
OS: 44.62 @ 180; 44.25 @ 090   (no inferior steepening)

Biomicroscopy

Both lenses were positioned superocentrally after the blink, with 2 to 3 mm of lens movement. In the left eye the conjunctival bleb had proliferated, expanding across the limbus and resting 0.5 mm on the cornea between 12 and 1 o'clock. It was also mildly vascularized, with superficial vessels. The left contact lens appeared to periodically rub against the leading edge of the bleb. Fluorescein revealed mild apical alignment, no staining or SPK on the right cornea, but moderate mid-peripheral corneal staining between 9 and 11 o'clock and mild linear staining of the anterior edge of the bleb overlapping the lens (Plate 25, *A*). The stain in the left eye crossed over a vessel close to the bleb surface. The patient was instructed to temporarily discontinue left contact lens wear and was given artificial tears for use qid along with a preservative-free topical lubricating ointment to use at bedtime (OS).

Ophthalmological consultation about this bleb determined that expansion had occurred; however, because of her long-standing low IOP without drugs, it was thought any excision of the bleb would be unwarranted given the potential risks. Due to the progression of the bleb in the left eye, it was decided to decrease the lens diameter in an effort to minimize bleb/lens edge interaction.

New left contact lens prescription

	BCR/SCR/PCR	Power	OAD/OZD	CT
OS:	7.64/10.0/12.0 mm	+6.50 D	8.4/7.4	0.35 mm

The laboratory was advised to carefully round off the edge. The material was Boston Equalens, and the design single cut. At the follow-up/dispensing visit 8 days later:

Visual acuity with RGPs

OD: 20/30
OS: 20/50

Keratometry

OD: 46.12 @ 150; 46.75 @ 060   (no inferior steepening)
OS: 44.50 @ 180; 44.12 @ 090   (no inferior steepening)

Biomicroscopy

Lens positioning in the right eye was superocentral with the blink and demonstrated 2 mm of movement. Lens positioning in the left eye was also superocentral after blinking, with 3 mm of vertical movement not in contact with the bleb edge. A separation of 0.5 mm existed between the bleb edge and the lens edge, as shown in Plate 25, B. Fluorescein revealed mild apical alignment of the right and left lenses, with moderate edge lift of the left. The patient continues to uneventfully wear the smaller-diameter left contact lens without any further incidence of pain or bleeding.

III. Assessment/Plan

This unusual case demonstrates that in post-surgical follow-up care, glaucoma patients with filtering blebs can successfully wear RGP contact lenses yet may also experience edge encroachment problems. Eye irritation, pain, and/or mild bleeding are landmark symptoms and clinical signs for contact lens practitioners to consider when fitting bleb patients into RGPs. Lens materials that contain UV absorbers are mandatory with any aphakic patient wearing such lenses. A list of RGP-UV absorbing materials is given in the box. Due to the superficial nature of vascularization on the bleb surface, mild laceration of the vessel by the lens edge caused by impingement, sharpness, or friction would have been inevitable with a larger-diameter lens.

IV. Alternative Management Plan/Summary

Options for the patient with a filtering bleb who wears contact lenses are limited. Because of the inevitable lens edge overlap with the bleb,

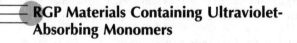

RGP Materials Containing Ultraviolet-Absorbing Monomers

Boston 7
Envision
Equalens I, Equalens II
Fluoroperm 30, 60, 92
RXD I

soft lenses are not really suitable. Hydrogel lenses are too large. RGPs are an option if there is careful follow-up to monitor for expansion of the bleb onto the cornea, a recognized postoperative complication.[14] Bleb encroachment onto the cornea is thought to be due to the massaging-down effect of the upper lid on the bleb. If bleb expansion becomes problematic, surgical adjustment can be performed. As a precaution against bleb/lens edge friction, clinicians are advised to encourage their patients to routinely use copious amounts of artificial tears with nightly lubricating ointment installation, especially in difficult cases such as this, in which the bleb has encroached onto the cornea.

• Case Five: Resistant Giant Papillary Conjunctivitis (GPC)

I. Subjective Data

A 26-year-old woman presented with an aggravated case of giant papillary conjunctivitis (GPC) that had been resistant to efforts to control it by several practitioners. She had worn extended-wear soft lenses for 8 years (5 in a single pair and 3 in 2-week disposables). Previous attempts to manage the GPC had included changing to a deposit-resistant material (CSI-T), converting to disposable soft lenses, and increasing enzyme treatment frequency to twice a week. After each change, she experienced temporary (3- to 6-month) relief followed by a rebound of the GPC. Because she was a flight attendant, she needed extended-wear lens capability and a disinfection system that would be simple and easy to use. She preferred the ReNu Multipurpose solution for disinfection but did not regularly use an enzyme treatment. She frequently rubbed her eyes when they itched and she reported pulling "strands of mucus junk" out of them every morning.

II. Objective Data

Visual acuity with disposable lenses

OD: 20/25
OS: 20/25-1

Overrefraction

OD: −0.25 D   (20/20)
OS: −0.25 D   (20/20-1)

Current contact lens prescription

	BCR	OAD	Power
OD: Acuvue	8.8 mm	14.0 mm	−3.50 D
OS: Acuvue	8.8 mm	14.0 mm	−4.00 D

Manifest refraction

OD: −3.75 DS   (20/20)
OS: −4.25 −0.25 × 160   (20/20)

Keratometry

OD: 43.75 @ 180; 44.12 @90   (mires slightly blurred)
OS: 43.37 @ 160; 43.81 @70   (mires moderately blurred)

Biomicroscopy

The right disposable lens was centrally positioned and had 1.0 mm of movement with blinking. The left lens was centrally positioned, with barely noticeable movement (less than 0.5 mm). There was mild palpebral conjunctival heaping adjacent to and slightly overlapping each lens edge, and both lenses demonstrated a significant amount of proteinlike deposit plaque (Plate 26). Without the lenses the right eye had moderate hyperemia of the superior and inferior palpebral conjunctivae, 1.50 mm round superior and 1.00 mm round inferior palpebral conjunctival papillae, and mild diffuse bulbar conjunctival hyperemia. The left eye had moderate hyperemia of the superior and inferior palpebral conjunctivae, 1.75 mm round superior and 1.25 mm round inferior palpebral conjunctival papillae with roughened surface apices, and moderate bulbar conjunctival hyperemia. Fluorescein revealed unstable tear film spreading across both corneas with a tear break-up time (B.U.T.) of 9 seconds in the right eye and 6 seconds in the left. Both corneas also had a mild diffuse superficial punctate keratitis with dustlike pattern. Short (less than 2 mm) strands of mucus were present in both inferior cul-de-sacs.

The patient was instructed to discontinue extended wear and switch to daily wear. Although her present 2-week Acuvue lenses were adequate for daily wear, we suggested that she switch from ReNu Multipurpose to AOSept disinfection. We also requested that she use Ultrazyme enzyme treatment every seventh day so as to minimize an apparent accelerated protein build-up. A new pair of lenses was issued with updated lens powers:

	BCR	OAD	Power	
OD:	Acuvue	8.8 mm	14.0 mm	−3.75 D	(20/20)
OS:	Acuvue	8.8 mm	14.0 mm	−4.25 D	(20/20-1)

She was asked to return to our office in 2 weeks. Six weeks later (after she had rescheduled the visit three times, due to her hectic flight/travel schedule) she reported improved overall eye comfort, with less itching, but she continued to have mucus strands in the morning in both medial canthi. However, she had been able to refrain from extended wear despite her rigorous travel schedule. She was distressed about the ongoing mucus problem, in that it embarrassed her when passengers would notice dried accumulations around her eyes. Thus she was in need of a quick solution—both because of her time restrictions in attending follow-up visits and because she had frequent contact with the public.

Visual acuity with 1-day-old Acuvue

OD: 20/20
OS: 20/20

Overrefraction

OD: Plano
OS: Plano

Keratometry

OD: 43.62 @ 180; 44.00 @ 090　　(mires slightly blurred)
OS: 43.25 @ 160; 43.76 @ 070　　(mires slightly blurred)

Biomicroscopy

With the disposables on both eyes there was bilateral central position-ing with 0.25 mm movement upon blinking. Previously noted con-junctival heaping over the edge of the left lens was absent. Both lens surfaces displayed a mild grayish hazy film that did not appear to cause any hydrophobic spotting. Without the lenses her palpebral conjunctiva demonstrated papillae (OD 1.0 mm superior and 0.75 mm inferior, OS 1.5 mm superior and 1.0 mm inferior). There was a mild palpebral conjunctival hyperemia of the upper and lower lids of both eyes. Mucus strands were detected in the inferior cul-de-sac of the left eye. Fluorescein demonstrated continued, though slightly improved, tear B.U.T.s (10 seconds OD, 7 seconds OS).

Because of her difficult schedule, it was decided to augment her management with enzyme cleaning every 3 days and Opticrom 4% to be used qid for 1 month, tid for 1 month, and then bid for mainte-nance. She received her Opticrom at a hospital pharmacy from a sterile transfer of Nasalcrom into a sterile ophthalmic dropper bottle. She was instructed to continue daily wear only and to use rewetting drops whenever flying to irrigate and rehydrate the lenses. Subsequent follow-up visits revealed sustained comfort, very little itching (except on international flights), a dramatic drop in mucus strand formation, and a pinkish color of the palpebral conjunctiva with only random papillae of less than 0.25 mm circumference. She also reported rapid deterioration with resulting symptoms if she tried to eliminate either her frequent enzyme treatments or her Opticrom dosing.

III. Assessment/Plan

Although a devoted contact lens wearer, this patient was adversely affected by her occupational environment. Clinicians who are manag-ing patients in similar corneal desiccation-inducing environments (such as shopping malls or frequent computer use) need to forewarn their patients that the work environment may be a major limitation to achieving full-time contact lens wear. Because this patient was exposed to dry air, smoke, and closed ventilation for long periods, she was especially penalized as a contact lens wearer. However, by being flexible and willing to try different lens-cleaning and ocular medication techniques, she was able to ultimately adapt to her environment with overall success.

IV. Alternative Management Plan/Summary

Patients with GPC can be difficult to please and manage unless clinicians and patients are sometimes willing to accept a combination treatment approach.[3] Although traditional treatment for GPC has been directed at modifying wearing time, changing materials, and using the least preserved solutions available, supplemental treatment with topical antihistamines, mast cell stabilizers,[1] or nonsteroidal antiinflammatory drugs is quietly but effectively becoming a preferred approach in difficult-to-manage cases. A careful evaluation of the occupational environment may reveal contributing factors (such as dust or vapor, dehumidified air, and/or allergen-borne debris) that can, singly or collectively, prevent a patient from wearing contact lenses at work. Therapeutic agents that may alter the allergic response to environmental irritants are listed in the box.

Pharmacological Agents for Ocular Allergies

Vasoconstrictor/antihistamine combinations
  Albalon A
  Naphcon A
  Opcon A
  Prefrin A
  Vasocon A
Topical antihistamines
  Livostin
Mast cell stabilizers
  Alomide
  Opticrom
Topical nonsteroidal antiinflammatories
  Acular
  Ocufen
  Profenal
  Voltaren

CLINICAL PEARL

A careful evaluation of the occupational environment may reveal contributing factors (such as dust or vapor, dehumidified air, and/or allergen-borne debris) that can, singly or collectively, prevent a patient from wearing contact lenses at work.

• Case Six: Asymptomatic On-Eye RGP Lens Fracture

I. Subjective Data

A 47-year-old man who was a full-time Tangent Streak bifocal contact lens wearer returned to the office for a routine eye examination. He had no complaints about his lenses and had successfully worn them for 17 years (10 years PMMA, 7 years various RGPs). However, he had a long history of smeary vision resulting from any exposure to smoke. His medical history was unremarkable except for mild allergies and a small amount of bilateral amblyopia. He used the Boston Advance solution system combined with once-a-week Pro Free enzyme treatment to manage a persistent protein plaque buildup.

II. Objective Data

Visual acuity with Tangent Streak bifocals

OD: 20/25+2 (J1)
OS: 20/25+2 (J1)

Overrefraction

OD: No improvement
OS: No improvement

Currently worn contact lenses

	BCR	Power	OAD	OZD
OD: Tangent Streak bifocals, single-cut design	−7.94 mm	−4.00/+2.25 D	9.4×9.0 mm	7.8 mm
OS: Tangent Streak bifocals, single-cut design	−7.94 mm	−3.50/+2.25 D	9.4×9.0 mm	7.8 mm

	Prism	Seg height	SCR (W)	PCR(W)
OD:	3 Δ	3.9 mm	9.50(0.4 mm)	11.50(0.4 mm)
OS:	3 Δ	3.9 mm	9.50(0.4 mm)	11.50(0.4 mm)

Manifest refraction

OD: −3.50 −0.25 × 160   (20/25+2)
OS: −3.50 −1.00 × 180   (20/25+2)
    Add: +2.00 @ 16 inches   OU
    +2.25 @ 14 inches   OU*

Keratometry

OD: 44.00 @ 160; 42.37 @ 070   (smooth mires)
OS: 44.12 @ 180; 42.50 @ 090   (smooth mires)

Biomicroscopy

With the Tangent Streak bifocal lenses on both eyes there was central to inferior positioning with a rapid lens drop after each blink. The right lens had 3 to 4 mm of vertical movement with a horizontal orientation. Its thicker inferior truncated edge rested gently on the inferior limbus, with slight (0.5 mm) limbal encroachment. This lens also displayed an enormous arclike fracture from the superior edge that extended down to the segment line. The fracture was subtle when viewed by conventional illumination (Plate 27, A) but was easily visualized by indirect retro-illumination, as shown in Plate 27, B. There was also a moderate amount of anterior lens surface hazing. The lens was easily removed with a DMV plunger. Without the right lens on the eye, fluorescein staining revealed mild nasal and temporal punctate staining but no apposition of the stain to the fracture line.

The left lens was central to inferior after each blink, with a similar inferior corneal resting position that also crossed the limbus. Lens movement with the blink was 4 to 5 mm. The segment orientation was horizontal, and the lens appeared to be physically intact. Fluorescein installation with the lens on the eye revealed central apical alignment, mild 180° midperipheral bearing, and a low edge lift. After the lens had been removed, there was mild nasal and temporal staining with a trace amount of arclike inferior stain coincident with the rocking motion of the truncated inferior edge.

The patient was completely unaware of the lens fracture. He reported no prior right lens awareness or sharpness. However, he revealed, under careful questioning, that his cleaning technique was to vigorously rub both lenses between his fingers, just as he had always done when cleaning his old PMMA lenses. This occurred despite previous lens-handling instructions and reminders to the contrary. It should also be noted that the right lens broke into two pieces as it was being removed from the DMV suction cup. The patient was asked to abandon contact lens wear until a new right replacement lens could be ordered and received. Since he had a pair of wearable spectacles to rely

---

*The patient's habitual working distance was 14 inches.

on during the interim, he was able to comfortably wait until the replacement arrived.

At follow-up and dispensing of the right lens 6 days later, a comprehensive patient reeducation effort in Tangent Streak bifocal handling was performed. The patient was able to demonstrate his understanding by first cleaning a diagnostic lens and then his old left lens and the new right one. After acknowledging the correct RGP handling techniques (see Assessment/Plan), which were notably different from his PMMA experiences, he was given the lenses.

Visual acuity with the new contact lenses

OD: 20/25+3　　(J1 @ 14 inches)
OS: 20/25+3　　(J1 @ 14 inches)

Overrefraction

OD: No improvement
OS: No improvement

Keratometry

OD: 43.87 @ 160; 42.25 @ 070　　(smooth mires)
OS: 44.00 @ 180; 42.37 @ 090　　(smooth mires)

Biomicroscopy

The right lens demonstrated central to inferior positioning with 4 mm of vertical movement after each blink. The inferior lens edge came to rest on the lower limbus. The left lens demonstrated the same characteristics except that the segment height was 0.5 mm below the inferior pupil margin. Fluorescein revealed bilateral apical alignment, 100° midperipheral bearing, and a moderate edge clearance (except inferiorly, where it was low). The Tangent Streak lenses were dispensed, and subsequent follow-up visits were uneventful in terms of lens breakage or loss. In an effort to inhibit accelerated protein buildup, the patient was instructed to increase his enzyme treatment to two times per week.

III. Assessment/Plan

Current RGP handling techniques[8] recommend cleaning the lens with a back-and-forth motion in the palm of the hand using the fifth finger. This patient's lens fracture was the result of overzealous handling and was characteristic of many PMMA wearers, who are accustomed to vigorous finger rubbing as a means of *scrubbing* their lenses clean. Also Tangent Streak bifocal lenses are essentially single-cut designs that result in an ultrathin (0.19 mm) superior and an ultra thick (0.40 mm) inferior (prism-ballast) lens profile.

This disparity between superior and inferior edge thicknesses, further aggravated by an absence of thickness-equalizing lenticular design, can be a recipe for lens breakage when conventional PMMA handling techniques are used. In addition, this patient was motivated to rub his lenses harder in the mistaken belief that aggressive cleaning would rid him of his "smeary" vision.

IV. Alternative Management Plan/Summary

Clinicians fitting the Tangent Streak bifocal need to be aware that the design is not available in a stability-enhancing lenticular carrier. Therefore greater caution needs to be exercised when handling these single-cut lenses. An alarming (inadvertent) potential for large minus repowering has been demonstrated when patients continually rub their lenses with an abrasive cleaner. This abrasive/handling thinning effect increases with time, precariously reducing the central lens thickness and consequently increasing the minus power. With proper initial instruction, most lens fractures can be avoided. If repeat fractures or breakages occur, it may be advisable to consider other lens designs as a means of minimizing replacement costs. Other presbyopia designs could include (1) different alternating bifocals, (2) simultaneous vision, or (3) monovision.

As former PMMA wearers appear to exhibit improved wearing success, it is vital that handling reinstruction become an essential part of the dispensing process.[8]

• Case Seven: Radial Compression Keratopathy

I. Subjective Data

A 22-year-old woman wearing 2½-year-old daily-wear lenses on a flexible-wear basis presented to the office for the first time with complaints of bilateral "eye aching," redness, hazy vision (especially around headlights at night), and a "tightness" sensation when her lenses are removed. She admitted to occasionally using her "cleaning" (disinfection) solution but noticed her eyes had been stinging upon lens insertion. She stated that her solution container had a "pewter ring" (AODISC Neutralizer) on the bottom that was "supposed to be changed about once a year"; she could not recall when she had last changed the disc. She also recalled a "pill" she was to be using, perhaps once a month. She discontinued this, however, because when she used it the first time it fizzled and foamed. Upon further questioning, she stated she had received her lenses at a commercial optical mall and had informed the staff person that she was a new, inexperienced wearer. She was given her lenses and care kit and told to practice at home and to call if there were any problems. Her medical history was unremarkable, her ocular history negative, and she denied having any history of glaucoma or amblyopia.

II. Objective Data

Visual acuity with present hydrogel contact lenses:

OD: 20/30+2
OS: 20/30–3

Overrefraction

OD: –0.75 D (20/25)
OS: –0.50 D (20/25)

Currently worn hydrogel lenses

	BCR/Power	OAD	
OD:	Brand unidentifiable	Unreadable	Approximately 13.5 mm
OS:	Brand unidentifiable	Unreadable	Approximately 13.5 mm

Keratometry (within 2 minutes of removal)

OD: 41.62 @ 020; 42.12 @ 110   (mires very blurry)
OS: 41.50 @ 175; 41.75 @ 85   (mires even blurrier)

Klein keratoscope (within 5 minutes of removal)

OD: Ring patterns have blurry edges; no unusual steepening or flattening
OS: Ring patterns appear spotty, with isolated disseminated areas of gross distortion; no significant steepening or flattening

Manifest refraction (within 10 minutes of removal)

OD: –4.75 –0.75 × 20   (20/25)
OS: –5.25 –0.50 × 175   (20/25-2)

Biomicroscopy

With hydrogel lenses on, the findings were remarkably similar in both eyes: diffuse moderate conjunctival hyperemia in a thin band-like pattern adjacent to the lens edges, which appeared to indent the conjunctiva slightly (Plate 28,*A*). Both lenses were centered but displayed no gross or localized movement, even after vigorous blinking. After lens removal, the right cornea displayed a 300° quasi-circumferential series of gray epithelial mounds, side by side and perpendicular to the limbus, approximately 0.25 mm wide and 0.75 to 1.50 mm in length. The left cornea also displayed a similar side-by-side intralimbal epithelial mounding, which in some cases overlapped onto the limbus. The midperipheral and peripheral corneas were mildly edematous. With fluorescein instilled, both showed areas of epithelial mounding with significant fluorescein uptake. After irrigation the staining persisted in the same areas and with similar density and intensity (Plate 28, *B*).

Lid eversion revealed bilateral upper and lower hyperemia with papillae that were approximately 0.25 mm inferiorly and 0.5 mm superiorly. Some mucus was present in the nasal canthi. The patient was diagnosed with radial compression keratopathy secondary to (an assumed) base curve radius steepening and diameter reduction. Although her records were unavailable, she stated that her first 18 months of soft lens wear had been uneventful. Only in the last 6 months could she recall her symptoms increasing. To control and reverse her edema and hyperemia, she was instructed to discontinue all hydrogel lens wear for 10 days. She was also asked to instill Muro 128 qid for 7 days and to place cold compresses over both eyes for 7 days. She was to allow 2 hours between use of the drops and to return within 1 week. The critical need for compliance to achieve improvement was emphasized.

At the follow-up visit 10 days later she was feeling significantly better. There was no more eye aching or tightness, and headlights had returned to their normal appearance. Also her eyes seemed less red. Since she was alarmed by her findings at the last examination, she had been conscientiously using her drops as directed.

Visual acuity with spectacles

OD: 20/20-2
OS: 20/20-3

Overrefraction

OD: −0.25 D   (20/20)
OS: −0.50 D   (20/20)

Keratometry

OD: 41.50 @ 020; 42.00 @ 110   (smooth mires)
OS: 41.50 @ 175; 42.12 @ 085   (smooth mires)

Klein keratoscope:

OD: Concentric rings clear; no abnormal steepening or flattening
OS: Concentric rings clear; no abnormal steepening or flattening

Manifest refraction

OD: −4.50 −0.25 × 020   (20/20+4)
OS: −5.00 −0.50 × 175   (20/20+4)

Biomicroscopy

Without any hydrogel lens wear for 10 days, the conjunctivae appeared to be clear, free of edema, and nonelevated. The corneas were smooth, without epithelial elevations or mounding, and were free of midperipheral or peripheral edema. After fluorescein was instilled, both the corneas and the conjunctivae appeared free of any uptake. The lids were everted and demonstrated a pinkish hue, with nonhyperemic papillae. No mucus strands were present in either canthus.

The patient was informed of her marked improvement, resulting from her careful compliance with instructions, and was successfully refitted with disposable soft lenses.

		BCR	OAD	Power	
OD:	Seequence II	9.0 mm	14.0 mm	−4.50 D	(20/20)
OS:	Seequence II	9.0 mm	14.0 mm	−5.00 D	(20/20-2)

She was asked to wear her hydrogel lenses only for daily wear, not for flexible or extended wear. She was also instructed in the proper use of AOSept disinfection. She was to discard the disk every 3 months and to use Ultrazyme after 7 days of routine daily wear. She has since progressed to 16 hours per day lens wear without any recurrence of hyperemia, GPC, or hydrogen peroxide irritation.

III. Assessment/Plan

Original records were not available, but this case was assumed to be an example of *aging hydrogel dehydration* that resulted in
(1) base curve radius steepening,
(2) diameter shrinkage,
(3) peripheral edge contraction, and
(4) reduction in oxygen supply to the cornea.
All these lens parameter changes can be directly or indirectly altered by lens water loss. This patient was (fortunately) successful because of her high motivation and renewed efforts at compliance. This is usually the case. After an initial assertion of compliance, patients often become lackadaisical and drift into noncompliance. With prior giant papillary conjunctivitis there may be a quick rebound if enzyme use is reduced or discontinued. Another factor contributing to the success of this patient was reeducation in the merits and proper use of the disinfection system. Lack of or incomplete hydrogen peroxide deactivation can create symptoms of stinging and/or redness. However, this is most often associated with improper use of the product. When properly used, hydrogen peroxide and the accompanying enzyme treatment are very effective.

IV. Alternative Management Plan/Summary

Several conditions can mimic radial compression keratopathy. Although the keratopathy is symptomatic, an asymptomatic (and perhaps antecedent) version, presenting as furrow staining, can occur. Extended wear is also strongly associated with furrow staining. In addition, limbal hypertrophy, of physically similar appearance, which is differentiated by its fluorescein disappearance with irrigation, can occur. A summary of these conditions appears in Table 9-2.

Although clinicians usually see edema in the central cornea, midperipheral and peripheral edema may also occur. The careful use of hypertonic agents available in 2% or 5% concentrations of sodium chloride can rapidly improve most cases, 2% being for mild and 5% for moderate or chronic edema. These agents act quickly in hypoxia-driven

TABLE 9-2

Differentiating Soft Contact Lens–Induced Corneal and Conjunctival Staining

Condition*	Fluorescein Symptoms	Pooling only	Persistent after irrigation
Radial compression keratopathy	Yes	No	Yes
Furrow staining	No	No	Yes
Limbal hypertrophy	No	Yes	No

*All three conditions may occur with (1) daily flexible- or extended-wear lenses, (2) single-pair soft lenses, and (3) disposable soft lenses.

intraepithelial edema, as opposed to interepithelial edema, which is associated with endothelial compromise and requires greater concentrations of hyperosmotic agents.[6] Ocular decongestants—for example, naphazoline hydrochloride, phenylephrine hydrochloride, and tetrahydrozaline hydrochloride[13]—may also be considered in cases with combined redness and edema.

To differentiate hypoxia-induced edema occurring independently of hyperemia, as opposed to preservative-induced edema and hyperemia, clinicians may want to begin with a single hypertonic product. If improvement does not occur, decongestants should be considered. Diffuse staining will occur in preservative-induced cases. There may be, in the future, significant improvements in hydrogel lens materials. If materials with high and super-high Dk/L ranges become approved by the Food & Drug Administration, clinicians may enjoy a rebound in hydrogel-prescribing opportunities for problem-prone cases (such as extended or flexible wear, impaired corneal physiology, and therapeutic bandage applications). Clearly, the "optimization of oxygenation" as suggested by Benjamin[4] offers our best hope in managing difficult cases and in providing a wider margin of safety for normal cases.

Summary

The management of contact lens–induced complications can be both challenging and frustrating but ultimately is the most rewarding clinical encounter that contact lens practitioners will face. Like detectives, clinicians must investigate a variety of clues, motivations, and contradictions. By segregating and separately evaluating patient history, lens materials, solutions, and compliance habits, clinicians will find the pursuit of complication etiology to be exciting and professionally satisfying.

Bibliography

1. Allansmith MR, Ross RN: Ocular allergy and mast cell stabilizers, *Surv Ophthalmol* 30:229-244, 1986.
2. Arffa RC: *Diseases of the cornea*, St Louis, 1991, Mosby, pp 164-192.
3. Begley CG: Giant papillary conjunctivitis. In Tomlinson A: *Complications of contact lens wear*, St Louis, 1992, Mosby, pp 237-252.
4. Benjamin WJ: Optimization of oxygenation: a water content "rule of thumb," *Int Contact Lens Clin* 20(3,4):61-64, 1993.
5. Carrell BA, Bennett ES, Henry VA, Grohe RM: The effect of rigid gas permeable lens cleaners on lens parameter stability, *J Am Optum Assoc* 63:193-200, 1992.
6. Chandler JW, Sugar J, Edelhauser HF: *External diseases: cornea, sclera, eyelids, lacrimal system*, St Louis, 1994, Mosby.
7. Dunn JP, Mondino BJ, Weissman BA: Infectitious keratitis in contact lens wearers. In Bennett ES, Weissman BA: *Clinical contact lens practice*, Philadelphia, 1991, JB Lippincott, Chapter 64.
8. Grohe RM: RGP problem solving, *Contact Lens Spectrum* 5:82-99, 1990.
9. Grohe RM, Lebow KA: Vascularized limbal keratitis, *Int Contact Lens Clin* 16(7,8):197-209, 1989.
10. Kaufman HE, Barron BA, McDonald MB, Waltman SR: *The cornea*, New York, 1988, Churchill-Livingston, pp 189-331.
11. Korb DR, Korb JME: Corneal staining prior to contact lens wear, *J Am Optum Assoc* 41:2-6, 1970.
12. Lebow KA: Clinical evaluation of the Boston Equalens for cosmetic extended wear, *Contact Lens Spectrum* 2:47-52, 1987.
13. *Physicians desk reference for ophthalmology*, Montvale, NJ, 1994, Medical Economics, 13-14.
14. Shields MB: *Textbook of glaucoma*, Baltimore, 1987, Williams & Wilkins, pp 461-479.
15. Stein RM, Clinch TE, Cohen EJ, et al: Infected vs sterile corneal infiltrates in contact lens wearers, *Am J Ophthalmol* 105:632-636, 1988.
16. Turner FD, Gower LA, Stein JM, et al: Compliance and contact lens care: a new assessment method, *Am J Ophthalmol Vis Sci* 70:998-1004, 1993.

Index